WORKING WITH CHILDREN
WITH SEXUAL BEHAVIOR PROBLEMS

Also from Eliana Gil

Books

Cultural Issues in Play Therapy
Eliana Gil and Athena A. Drewes, Editors

*The Healing Power of Play:
Working with Abused Children*
Eliana Gil

*Helping Abused and Traumatized Children:
Integrating Directive and Nondirective Approaches*
Eliana Gil

Play in Family Therapy
Eliana Gil

Treating Abused Adolescents
Eliana Gil

*Working with Children to Heal Interpersonal Trauma:
The Power of Play*
Eliana Gil

DVDs

Essentials of Play Therapy with Abused Children
Eliana Gil

Play Therapy for Severe Psychological Trauma
Eliana Gil

Working with Children with Sexual Behavior Problems

ELIANA GIL
JENNIFER A. SHAW

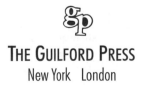

THE GUILFORD PRESS
New York   London

© 2014 The Guilford Press
A Division of Guilford Publications, Inc.
72 Spring Street, New York, NY 10012

www.guilford.com

Printed in the United States of America

This book is printed on acid-free paper.

Last digit is print number: 9 8 7 6 5 4 3 2 1

The authors have checked with sources believed to be reliable in their efforts to provide
information that is complete and generally in accord with the standards of practice that
are accepted at the time of publication. However, in view of the possibility of human error
or changes in behavioral, mental health, or medical sciences, neither the authors, nor the
editor and publisher, nor any other party who has been involved in the preparation or
publication of this work warrants that the information contained herein is in every respect
accurate or complete, and they are not responsible for any errors or omissions or the
results obtained from the use of such information. Readers are encouraged to confirm the
information contained in this book with other sources.

Library of Congress Cataloging-in-Publication Data

Gil, Eliana.
  Working with children with sexual behavior problems / by Eliana Gil and
Jennifer A. Shaw.
     pages cm
  Includes bibliographical references and index.
  ISBN 978-1-4625-1197-6 (cloth : alk. paper)
  1. Psychosexual disorders in children.   2. Children and sex.   3. Children—Sexual
behavior.   4. Child sexual abuse.   I. Shaw, Jennifer A.   II. Title.
  RJ506.P72G553 2014
  618.92′8583—dc23
                                                              2013016494

About the Authors

Eliana Gil, PhD, is senior partner in a private group practice, the Gil Institute for Trauma Recovery and Education in Fairfax, Virginia, which provides therapy, consulting, and training services. She is also Director of Starbright Training Institute for Child and Family Play Therapy in northern Virginia, where she provides multiple-day trainings on family play therapy and specialized therapy with youth (and their families) who have experienced childhood trauma. Dr. Gil has worked in the field of child abuse prevention and treatment for almost 40 years. In the last two decades she has directed two child sexual abuse treatment programs in northern Virginia (at Inova Kellar Center and Childhelp Children's Center of Virginia). She is a licensed marriage, family, and child counselor; an approved marriage and family therapy supervisor; a registered play therapist; and a registered play therapy supervisor. Dr. Gil also consults and trains across the United States and is an adjunct faculty member in Virginia Tech's Marriage and Family Therapy Department. She has served on the Board of Directors of the American Professional Society on the Abuse of Children and the National Resource Center on Child Sexual Abuse; she is also a former president of the Association for Play Therapy. Dr. Gil is the author of *The Healing Power of Play: Working with Abused Children; Play in Family Therapy; Treating Abused Adolescents; Helping Abused and Traumatized Children: Integrating Directive and Nondirective Approaches;* and other acclaimed books and video programs on child abuse and related topics. Many of her books have been translated into other languages, including Spanish. Originally from Guayaquil, Ecuador, Dr. Gil is bilingual and bicultural. She has three grandchildren under the age of 6.

Jennifer A. Shaw, PsyD, is a founding partner of the Gil Institute for Trauma Recovery and Education, and has worked in a number of clinical settings and capacities in metropolitan Washington, D.C. She provides individual, family, and group therapy to children and adolescents presenting with sexual behavior problems; with symptoms of depression, anxiety, and adjustment problems; and with complex trauma. She has been the coordinator of the specialized family-based program described in this book, the Boundary Project, in two clinical settings—at Childhelp Children's Center of Virginia and the Gil Institute for Trauma Recovery and Education. Dr. Shaw has also acquired specialized training and certification in conducting psychosexual risk assessments and treating sexual offending behaviors in adolescents and adults, and is currently working toward certification as a registered play therapist. She provides trainings at the local, regional, and state level for professionals who work with families of children with sexual behavior problems. Dr. Shaw has coauthored two book chapters with Dr. Gil. Their latest collaboration is a children's book entitled *A Book for Kids about Private Parts, Touching, Touching Problems, and Other Stuff.*

Preface

Although our interest in children with sexual behavior problems has spanned two decades, the questions remain the same: What is normative sexual play? What prompts children to develop sexual preoccupations? How do we know when such children need professional help? And, finally, in what circumstances is child-to-child sexual activity abusive or harmful?

In spite of myriad resources to help parents or other primary caregivers and professionals sort out these questions to their satisfaction, something still seems to get in the way. For some reason, accessible information is either dismissed or misunderstood. Even after parents, caregivers, and professionals search the Internet, locate the available information on this topic, and read voraciously, confusion can still persist. The reason for this, we believe, is that sexuality in general, and childhood sexuality in particular, still elicit a range of rational and irrational thoughts that often produce uncomfortable feelings; these thoughts and feelings then complicate the taking in and processing of information. When anxiety or fear enter the mix, primary caregivers and professionals alike can struggle to make sense of what is going on and how to respond.

This book was written to help professionals choose a variety of interventions when they are asked to evaluate a specific situation or make recommendations to parents and other caregivers. The first three chapters of the book discuss sexual behavior problems and note the progress that has been made in understanding the origins of these problems and contributing factors. Issues such as prior victimization, exposure to various media, the influence of social pressure, and factors influencing the merging of sex and aggression are explored. In Chapter Four, we discuss a child-friendly assessment process for helping children engage in honest conversations about their thoughts and feelings; in Chapter Five, we describe consensus-based areas for treatment and discuss our approaches to working with parents. In Chapter Six, we describe the Boundary Project—a program that Eliana Gil developed many years ago and that has since been implemented in a variety of treatment settings. Jennifer A. Shaw has spearheaded the Boundary Project since 2003 and has contributed greatly to its current form and shape. Pre- and posttreatment testing of this model shows a decrease in sexual behavior problems and an increase in healthier social functioning, according to parental reports, and other preliminary findings are likewise optimistic. In addition, the early chapters review many treatment efforts across the United States that also indicate positive treatment outcomes in programs with a cognitive-behavioral foundation. It appears that for children with sexual behavior problems, a combination of approaches to help them get better control of their impulses, thoughts, and feelings, along with assistance to parents in monitoring and supervising their children's behaviors, can be quite successful.

Chapters Seven through Ten are case studies that highlight how theory and practice inform our work. These case examples illustrate the high priority we give to eliciting the cooperation of parents or other caregivers in successfully implementing the treatment model and helping their children. Without this support, our work is much more challenging, and we encourage families to understand the critical contribution they make. These chapters also illustrate our integrated approach to working with young children with sexual behavior problems, demonstrating aspects of both assessment and treatment.

Contents

CHAPTER ONE

Children with Sexual Behavior Problems

An Introduction

Mental health professionals tasked with identifying, assessing, and addressing sexual behavior problems in young children (i.e., those below school age) and school-age children face unique and complex challenges, which have been increasingly recognized over the past two decades. Children with sexual behavior problems appear to be sexually preoccupied and overstimulated, and the behavioral manifestations are diverse and vary significantly in frequency, scope, and intensity. These manifestations can include both self-directed behaviors (such as excessive masturbation, disinhibited masturbation in public, and/or self-exposure) and other-directed behaviors (ranging from fondling to coercive sexual play to aggressive sexual abuse of other children). Many parents and other caregivers, and even many professionals, are uncomfortable with open discussions of childhood sexuality—especially overt sexual behaviors. Such behaviors are particularly distressing when they are observable outside the home. Adults' discomfort not only can interfere with accurate reporting of these children's behaviors over time, but may contribute to inappropriate and ineffective responses to the children, including rigid, extreme interventions focused on the safety of others. As Friedrich (2007) has noted,

> the automatic response to childhood sexuality is that it is problematic and reflective of a sexually abusive experience . . . and while it is true in some cases, it only explains a small percentage of children's

1

sexual behaviors. An option to our uncertainty is to step back, ana-lyze whether our perspective is appropriate, and then create a sensitive response. (p. 8)

Unfortunately for families of children with sexual behavior prob-lems, stereotypes often serve as reference points: The children are viewed as either victims of sexual abuse or future sex offenders. Neither stereo-type is accurate for the majority of these children, but such assump-tions can lead to repercussions that do not correspond to the children's actions (Friedrich, 2007). In the absence of an informed, individualized, and sensitive approach, many children are inaccurately labeled, stigma-tized at school, marginalized in community settings, and socially iso-lated, particularly in cases where more intrusive sexual behavior prob-lems place other children at risk. Misconceptions regarding etiology and prognosis can result in labeling young children as "juvenile offenders," which can provoke fear-based responses from parents or other caregiv-ers, as well as school personnel and after-school care providers. Inap-propriate, exaggerated, or generalized responses to behavioral problems alone can prohibit or delay interventions that address a child's or fam-ily's underlying conflicts. A misguided, limited, or exclusive focus on the sexual behavior problems can leave the child alone to cope with his or her internal conflicts, and the familial factors unexamined. Too often, children with sexual behavior problems are left untreated, and caregiv-ers are left without adequate support and appropriate guidance.

Sexual preoccupation and sexualized behaviors associated with overstimulation can be diminished when caregivers learn to use tools that are now known to address sexual behavior problems effectively, while also addressing the caregivers' and/or family's emotional needs. As research has increasingly confirmed, sexual behavior problems in young and school-age children can be successfully treated in a relatively short time by correcting misinformation and misperceptions through psy-choeducation for both caregivers and children, in combination with an integrative, family-focused approach by therapists trained to work with children and their families. With correct information, proven strategies to redirect behaviors, and consistent responses across a child's care set-tings, caregivers can confidently advocate for their child's mental health needs; compassionately respond to the child's unique emotional life; effectively address underlying familial issues that may have contributed to the emergence or maintenance of sexual behavior problems; and build or rebuild a healthy family system.

DEFINING SEXUAL BEHAVIOR PROBLEMS

Chaffin, Letourneau, and Silovsky (2002) have defined problematic sexual behaviors in childhood as follows: behaviors (1) that occur with unexpected frequency, in coercive contexts, or between youth in different age groups; and (2) that resist intervention, interfere with development, and/or are associated with emotional distress. The Association for the Treatment of Sexual Abusers (ATSA) Task Force on Children with Sexual Behavior Problems (Chaffin et al., 2006) more specifically defines children with sexual behavior problems as "children ages 12 and younger who initiate behaviors involving sexual body parts (i.e., genitals, anus, buttocks, or breasts) that are developmentally inappropriate or potentially harmful to themselves or others" (p. 3). For young children especially, however, sexual behavior problems may not be directly related to sexual gratification/stimulation, but rather to anxiety, curiosity/imitation, attempts to self-soothe, desires for attention, or other factors (Silovsky & Bonner, 2003b). Sexual behavior problems may be self-focused or other-focused, as noted above; other-focused behaviors appear to vary in the degree of mutuality or coercion, the types of sexual acts, and the potential for harm. "The most concerning . . . cases involve substantial age or developmental inequalities; more advanced sexual behaviors; aggression, force or coercion; and harm or the potential for harm" (Chaffin et al., 2006, pp. 3–4). Research over the past decade suggests that children with sexual behavior problems are a highly hetereogeneous group, with few characteristics to distinguish them from other children (Chaffin et al., 2002).

Current research does not suggest that sexual behavior problems involve distinct behavior subtypes; rather, they appear to involve ranges in severity and intensity of the behaviors. These behaviors are diverse, however, as are these children's demographics, socioeconomic factors, mental health status, maltreatment and victimization histories, and familial factors (Chaffin et al., 2006). Severe and frequent sexual behavior problems do appear to involve more coexisting social issues, family problems, and child mental health issues (Hall, Mathews, Pearce, Sarlo-McGarvey, & Gavin, 1996). Children with sexual behavior problems are also more diverse than adolescent sex offenders in the sense that the younger group includes a substantial number of young girls, whereas adolescent offenders are primarily males (Silovsky & Niec, 2002). Bonner, Walker, and Berliner (1999) explored sexual behavior problem subtypes based on specific types of behavior, but the data do not suggest either a behavioral profile or a clear pattern of any factors that might differentiate children with sexual behavior problems from other children (Chaffin et al., 2002).

Up-to-date incidence and prevalence rates of childhood sexual behavior problems are not available. However, recent years have seen an increasing number of referrals for such problems to child protective service agencies, juvenile services, and both outpatient and inpatient clinical settings. Whether this increase is due to an actual rise in the behaviors or an increase in awareness/reporting, or a combination of these factors, is not yet known (Chaffin et al., 2006). The incidence rates of non-normative sexual behaviors in children reported by Friedrich et al. (2001) suggest that the more extreme sexual behavior problems are relatively rare occurrences.

In developing and conducting research with the Child Sexual Behavior Inventory (CSBI), William N. Friedrich and colleagues have provided the most comprehensive empirical examinations of normative and non-normative sexual behaviors to date. The CSBI (Friedrich, 1997) is a 38-item parent report measure designed for children ages 2–12 that covers a wide range of sexual behaviors, including boundary problems, sexual knowledge, voyeuristic behaviors, exhibitionism, sexual intrusiveness, sexual interest, sexual anxiety, gender role behavior, and self-stimulation. Friedrich et al. (1998) found that the most frequently observed behaviors involved boundary problems, self-stimulation, and exhibitionism. The more intense other-focused or intrusive behaviors (i.e., oral sex, anal and/or vaginal penetration, fondling) were much less often reported by caregivers.

Approximately 20% of caregivers in this study endorsed sexual behaviors that were within age-appropriate limits and considered developmentally related (CRI). Friedrich et al. (1998)

> observed [that] sexual behaviors were inversely related to age, with overall frequency peaking at year five for both boys and girls and dropping off over the next seven years. There was again an increase in sexually related behaviors with the onset of adolescence with a shift to increased interest in the opposite sex beginning at age 10 through 12 years. Also, [there were] few gender differences in terms of frequency or types of sexual behaviors exhibited.

A high percentage of children with sexual behavior problems have histories of physical or sexual abuse, neglect, or witnessing of domestic violence (Chaffin et al., 2006; Friedrich, 2007). Other contributing factors include overstimulating or inappropriate environmental factors, such as access to pornography, access to inappropriate television and other media programming, or inappropriate modeling of privacy and sexuality by caregivers. Professionals remain mystified, frustrated, and often stymied by the question of how best to respond to these children and their families. Too often, clinical responses appear to be random and subjective, or to have been adapted from treatment models developed for adolescent or adult sexual offenders.

With appropriate treatment for children and their families, and with appropriate community and caregiver supports, children with sexual behavior problems are found to be at very low risk for committing future sex offenses. The ATSA Task Force (Chaffin et al., 2006) has concluded that children with sexual behavior problems are at "no greater long-term risk for future sex offenses than other clinic children (2%–3%)," and that they are "qualitatively different" from older adolescent and adult sexual offenders (p. 2). Policies, assessment protocols, and the majority of commonly used treatment approaches are therefore inappropriate. As highlighted by the ATSA Task Force (2006, p. 2), policies placing children on public sex offender registries or segregating children with [sexual behavior problems] may offer little or no actual community protection while subjecting children to potential stigma and social disadvantage.

A review of the literature strongly suggests that sexual behavior problems in young and school-age children are responsive to an integrative treatment approach that includes psychoeducation, cognitive-behavioral therapy (CBT), and active and direct participation of the children's primary caregivers. Treatments that are longer-term, intensive, and restrictive do not appear to be necessary for most childhood sexual behavior problems (Friedrich, 2007; Chaffin et al., 2006).

SYNOPSIS OF RESEARCH ON TREATMENT AND PREDICTIVE FACTORS

Research is increasingly informing clinicians about effective interventions for nonsexual behavior problems in childhood, many of which are similar to factors associated with sexual behavior problems (e.g., poor impulse control, dysregulation affecting all areas of development, maltreatment in early childhood, chronic family dysfunction, attachment issues in the parent–child relationship, poor parenting practices). Thus interventions for some general childhood behavior problems are also appropriate for issues underlying childhood sexual behavior problems. One distinguishing feature, however, might be the type and increased level of adult supervision required for children with sexual behavior problems. Studies of existing child-centered, play-based, and developmentally appropriate approaches to working with young children in therapy, combined with the rich, growing body of research on CBT interventions for children facing myriad social, emotional, and behavioral concerns, serve to ground and enrich the current research on effective, specific interventions for childhood sexual behavior problems.

In a randomized trial of 115 children ages 6–12 with documented sexual behavior problems, Pithers, Gray, Busconi, and Houchens (1998) had children and their families participate in 32 sessions of either expressive therapy or a group program based on relapse prevention. Both groups included psychoeducational and CBT components. Adapted from adult sex offender treatment models, the relapse prevention approach was more focused on identifying relapse-related factors and building a prevention team than was the expressive approach; the latter simply provided education about sexual behavior rules/boundaries, emotional management, and the effects of sexual abuse, and taught problem-solving and social skills (Araji, 1997). Children in both groups demonstrated improvement by the middle phase of treatment, although children with symptoms of traumatic stress seemed to improve more in the relapse prevention group (Pithers et al., 1998). At follow-up, improvements were found in both groups, and the groups did not differ significantly (Bonner & Fahey, 1998).

Bonner et al. (1999) have developed a group CBT model for children ages 6–12 with sexual behavior problems. Based on behavior modification principles and a teaching–learning model for group management, the structured time-limited curriculum emphasizes impulse control, cognitive rules, decision making, and education. The primary treatment foci include (1) helping children to acknowledge the inappropriate sexual behavior; (2) teaching sexual behavior rules; (3) improving the children's impulse control; (4) providing sex education; and (5) preventing further abuse of self and others. A separate manual, with similar topic areas, is provided to a co-occurring parent group intervention. Parents or caregivers are involved in both monitoring sexual behaviors and supervising children's activities, as well as learning strategies to reinforce basic impulse control skills.

Bonner et al. (1999) used this manualized approach in a randomized trial assigning children with sexual behavior problems to either the psychoeducational CBT group program or a 12-session play therapy group. Posttreatment measures suggested that both treatment groups demonstrated short-term reductions in both sexual and nonsexual behavior problems. However, at a 10-year follow-up, the group receiving the CBT intervention demonstrated significantly greater long-term reduction in sexually abusive behaviors, as indicated by the number of sexual abuse perpetrations and sexual offense arrests. Furthermore, children in the CBT group were found to have a rate of future sex offenses (2%) similar to that of children with attention-deficit/hyperactivity disorder (ADHD) or other behavior problems but without a co-occurring sexual behavior problem (3%). Preliminary data on the Bonner et al. 12-session CBT parent and child group intervention suggest that the risk of childhood sexual behavior problems' continuing into adolescence and adulthood can be reduced to baseline levels with appropriate short-term treatment (Chaffin et al., 2006).

Using a wait-list control design, Silovsky, Niec, Bard, and Hecht (2007) evaluated the efficacy of a 12-week group CBT program for preschoolers with sexual behavior problems, who were evaluated weekly throughout the wait-list and treatment periods. A reduction in sexual behavior problems seemed to be related to the passage of time or other factors associated with interventions for caregivers or child welfare interventions, such as increased supervision and reduction of contact with other children. However, Silovsky et al. (2007) also found that the improvement of the children with the highest frequency of sexual behavior problems was much more rapid once the CBT was initiated (Chaffin et al., 2006).

Stauffer and Deblinger (1996) examined children with sexual behavior problems who were receiving CBT for traumatic stress symptoms related to sexual abuse. They noted greater reductions during treatment than during a wait-list period, and these reductions seemed to be maintained at a 3-month follow-up. Pre- to posttreatment decreases in sexual behavior problems have also been reported among children in outpatient psychotherapy focused specifically on these concerns (Friedrich, Luecke, Beilke, & Place, 1992).

Friedrich, Davies, Feher, and Wright (2003) have proposed a four-component model of variables that seem to predict children at greatest risk of engaging in problematic sexual behaviors. Supported by their previous research, these four components are modeling of sexuality, family adversity, modeling of coercive behavior, and general child behavior. Sexual abuse is commonly associated with sexual behavior problems, but not all victims of such abuse develop these problems. Factors related to family functioning (particularly in regard to boundaries and sexuality) are important, and social factors such as poverty, family stress, and otherwise strained parent–child relationships appear to increase the risk for the emergence of sexual behavior problems. Maltreatment and family violence are highly correlated with sexual behavior problems, as are more generalized behavioral/mental health problems and social deficits.

This review of the literature suggests that no single causal factor can best explain or predict sexual behavior problems in children. The degree to which a child is vulnerable to developing problems derives from a complex interaction of factors related to the child, family, and social environment (Grant & Lundeberg, 2009). In cases of sexual abuse, the development of a problematic sexual behavior is not a universal consequence (most likely due in part to the widely variable nature of sexual abuse), but it continues to be a recognizable and frequent occurrence (Friedrich, 1997).

The growing body of research suggests that a reduction of sexual behavior problems in young children occurs naturally over time, but that this reduction is accelerated by short-term treatment of both the child and primary caregiver(s), and to some extent by early detection and appropriate adult intervention. Treatments focused on and structured around the specific sexual behaviors appear to have the best results to date, as do CBT-based interventions; however, research examining the effectiveness of other therapies, including an integrative model, remains largely unexplored. Studies of CBT approaches that focus on sexual behavior problems and that involve primary caregivers have showed these approaches to work better than unstructured approaches (supportive therapy, play therapy). These findings include improvements in both short-term and long-term officially reported sexual offenses. Furthermore, research suggests that treatment targeting sexual behavior problems while also addressing symptoms of traumatic stress, for children with both sets of problems, can be effective in ameliorating both symptom groups.

Overall, studies are confirming that successful treatment outcomes can be achieved and can help to decrease sexual behavior problems in young and school-age children, and that short-term outpatient treatment is effective with a broad range of sexual behavior problems, including highly aggressive behaviors in both boys and girls. Benefits of a short-term, structured approach are also reported among children who have experienced significant trauma, children with varying levels of comorbid mental health issues, and varying levels of family problems. Short-term or time-limited outpatient CBT is therefore suggested as the treatment of choice for childhood sexual behavior problems at this time. When this is provided in conjunction with parent or caregiver involvement, improvement can be observed more quickly and can yield longer-term recovery for the family. CBT may not be an appropriate treatment choice for severe cases or for children with severe comorbid problems.

Outpatient CBT is the most studied treatment for childhood sexual behavior problems to date. Research on types of treatments that do not rely on a CBT orientation continues to be needed, and, as noted by Chaffin et al. (2006), there are no controlled outcome studies testing interventions for children placed in inpatient or residential settings. Moreover, behavioral parent training or family therapy approaches have not been tested specifically for children with sexual behavior problems, although they do show promising results in treating nonsexual behavior problems.

THE ROLE OF CAREGIVERS IN TREATMENT

As caregivers play a critical role in creating a nurturing, safe, calm, and nonsexualized environment for children, a consistent theme across the current literature on childhood sexual behavior problems is an emphasis on involving parents or other primary caregivers in treatment (Friedrich, 2007; Silovsky et al., 2007). These adults may be biological parents, extended family members, foster parents, or others; in cases where primary caregivers may change, clinicians should consider including both the present and the potential future caregivers (e.g., foster-to-adoptive parents) in treatment. In many cases, a child's home environment may have actively contributed to the development and/or maintenance of the child's sexual behavior. For intervention to be effective, this environment has to be made safer/more stable, and contributing factors must be explored and adjusted. "In other cases, the home environment may not have contributed to the problem, but . . . caregiver involvement in treatment may still be critical for providing support and for implementing day-to-day aspects of the intervention plan" (Chaffin et al., 2006, p. 16).

Like interventions for serious nonsexual behavior problems in children, interventions for sexual behavior problems are most effective when they incorporate a focused, goal-directed approach; teach primary caregivers and teachers how to use practical behavior management strategies; and strengthen parent–child relationships (Patterson, Reid, & Eddy, 2002). Several approaches to parent involvement can be considered, including joint caregiver–child sessions, family play therapy, regular concurrent sessions with parents and children, and in-home or family therapy modalities. The group therapy approaches used by Bonner et al. (1999) and Pithers et al. (1998) in randomized trials both included parent involvement in the children's group and/or in a regular parents' group (Chaffin et al., 2006). However, research is currently limited to CBT-focused interventions in both the child and parent groups.

Children with severe sexual behavior problems typically have severely problematic parent–child attachment. Friedrich (2007) states:

> My goal is to remind all of us of the centrality of relationships in both the etiology and treatment of children with sexual behavior problems. These children first learn to relate in a disturbed manner, and subsequently use this model of relationships in their interactions with other children. Altering the first model of relating can make a difference in how these children will relate to others, and I believe this is the most efficacious form of intervention. (Friedrich, 2007, p. 4)

Lieberman and Van Horn (2008) propose that a child's attachments, or the primary emotional relationships with the parents or other caregivers, should be given a prominent role across different disciplines in assessing and treating mental health problems. Despite this need for attachment-focused work, current interventions remain individual in nature and focused on altering cognitions related to the child's sexual behavior (Friedrich, 2007). Regardless of the presenting problem, severity of the behavior, or risk/potential of harm to others, every young child has core needs for parental love, protection, and socialization. When these core needs are consistently met, the child's sense of self is organized around two largely unconscious assumptions: the trust that the parents are capable of raising the child well, and the conviction that the child deserves this care (Ainsworth, Blehar, Waters, & Wall, 1978; Bowlby, 1988). Lieberman and Van Horn (2008) state:

> Fears of abandonment, loss of love, body damage, and doing wrong always play a role in shaping the child's response to external threats. For this reason, helpful parental responses to the child's fears must

always include the implicit or explicit message that the child will not be abandoned, will continue to be loved, and will be protected from harm. (p. 11)

For parents of children with frequent, severe, and/or intrusive sexual behavior problems, providing consistent, empathic, and loving messages to their children can be extremely difficult and counterintuitive. And yet parents must strive to provide a secure base to their children, in order to optimize the children's health. Greenspan (2002) suggests that the most important attribute of a secure child is probably having enough trust in relationships to use them in times of stress to feel better and find solutions.

SUMMARY

Childhood sexuality is progressive from birth and develops both according to individual factors and in concert with family, ethnic, social, and cultural influences. The assessment and treatment of childhood sexual behavior problems requires an understanding of the biological and psychosocial factors determining children's sexual development, gender role, patterns of sexual arousal, cognitions and beliefs around sexuality, and integration of sexual and aggressive patterns of behavior (American Academy of Child and Adolescent Psychiatry, 1999). Our overarching philosophies about, family-focused approach to, and interventions specific to childhood sexual behavior problems (see Chapters Four, Five, and Six of this book) have been significantly influenced by the wealth of research and literature provided by Friedrich and his colleagues. Applying these principles and strategies requires a rich understanding of child development, child psychology, parent–child attachment, family theory and therapy, and the theoretical constructs of play therapy theory and practice. Friedrich (2007) asserts that

> a new set of perspectives is needed to understand children with sexual behavior problems. Paramount to this is a focus on attachment and relational issues in therapy. Sexually abused children are compelling, given their trauma, and command focus on the victimization experience and correcting the related impacts on affect and cognition. However, the larger attachment dynamics and family relations are often ignored, even though they are frequently the largest contributors to adjustment. (p. 4)

There is much reason to feel optimistic about our abilities to help children who develop sexual behavior problems, as well as their families. There appear to be no data suggesting a linear cause-and-effect relationship between such problems and later offending behaviors. The substantial work done to date is promising and provides guidelines for ongoing prevention of and intervention with this challenging problem, which elicits such varied responses.

CHAPTER TWO

Differentiating Normative Childhood Sexuality from Sexual Behavior Problems

Sarah, a 30-year-old mother, called to leave a frantic voice mail: "I'm really worried that something has happened to my daughter. All of a sudden, when she was kissing her dad good night, she asked him to stick his tongue in her mouth! I'm scared to death that something bad has happened to her!"

Steve, a 40-year-old father of five, called with the following worry: "I noticed it was really quiet last night, and I went in to check what the kids were up to. My boys were naked in bed together, and one of them had a hard-on! I need to know what's going on here. Please call me."

Dante, a 66-year-old grandfather, had a similar worry: "This boy is constantly touching the front of his pants, whether there's someone watching him or not. I want him to come into therapy to stop doing this strange behavior."

Another parent called, stating, "The school has just suspended my kindergartener for a week because he showed his private parts to another child! I'm in a panic, and I think he needs some help fast!"

These are typical concerns from parents and other caregivers who call mental health professionals to discuss what they perceive as problems in their children's behaviors—and yet some of the behaviors in these examples may or may not be reasons for parental concern. Numerous factors go into determining whether children are exhibiting normative sexual behaviors or whether the behaviors in question signal a need for assistance. In spite of the fact that many publications in various media have attempted to tackle the issue of normative versus non-normative sexual development, parents/other caregivers frequently seem challenged and overwhelmed when facing a situation that relates to their children's sexual behaviors. Mental health professionals may sometimes feel similarly baffled by what appear to be unusual sexual behaviors, and may feel unable to provide responses that take into account the myriad factors often accompanying true sexual behavior problems. Although research and other literature on this issue can seem difficult to obtain, the available literature does provide us with guidelines, reassurances, and suggestions.

Children with problematic sexual behaviors are first and foremost children (Silovsky, Swisher, Widdifield, & Burris, 2012)—who have a natural inclination for exploration and a need to test limits in order to achieve developmental milestones. Like all children, they learn what is OK and not OK from their caregivers and from things that happen in their environment. When something is confusing in their lives, they may act it out or play it out. When something is interesting or brings pleasure, they may be more inclined to repeat the action that brought pleasure. However, when events, situations, or people feel frightening to them or overwhelm their perceived capacity to cope, they can become dysregulated and develop novel behaviors that surprise or overwhelm their caretakers.

When there is damage to a child's basic relationship with a primary caregiver (the attachment bond), the child can become distressed and may manifest this distress in a variety of ways that get attention from adults. The primary need—to resolve the attachment damage—is often overlooked once the problem behavior is replaced by a more appropriate behavior. The underlying distress then finds other ways of interfering with healthy development.

The forms of normative childhood sexual interests and behaviors vary across development and across cultures (Friedrich et al., 2001). As suggested by Friedrich (2007), childhood sexuality is as much about child development as it is about family and social context:

> Simple answers about the appropriateness of a single behavior should be avoided, since the behavior in question typically did not emerge fully

articulated in the child's mind but required some combination of the child, the child's history, feelings at the time, opportunity, the social environment, behavioral repertoire, and the responses of adults. (p. 9)

An essential consideration in assessing a child with a possible sexual behavior problem, then, is to understand the problematic behaviors in the context of normative childhood sexual development, cultural influences, and environmental factors (Friedrich et al., 2001).

NORMATIVE SEXUAL BEHAVIORS

As one of us (Gil, 1993) stated, two things about childhood sexuality can be said with certainty: (1) Sexual curiosity, interest, experimentation, and behavior are progressive over time, and (2) sexual development is affected by a number of variables (p. 21). Normative sexual play is usually spontaneous, and includes pleasure, joy, laughter, embarrassment, and varying levels of inhibition and disinhibition (Araji, 1997). Like all aspects of a child's development, sexual development begins at birth and progresses though stages or phases. These stages can be seen both in sexual behaviors and in the acquisition of sexual knowledge (Friedrich et al., 1998; Friedrich, 2007). Sexual knowledge and behavior for any given child are influenced by the child's age, what the child observes, and what the child is taught directly (including cultural and religious beliefs about sexuality and sexual behaviors) (Friedrich et al., 1998; Friedrich, 2007). In addition, children nowadays get much of their education from the larger environment of the mass media, which we discuss in Chapter Three.

Friedrich's contribution to our ability to distinguish problematic from normative sexual behaviors cannot be overestimated. As we have noted in Chapter One, Friedrich and colleagues utilized the CSBI to establish a baseline for normative childhood sexual behaviors (Friedrich, Grambsch, Broughton, Kuiper, & Beilke, 1991; Friedrich et al., 1998, 2001). In so doing, they demonstrated that all children engage in sexual behaviors, thus debunking the myth that sexuality is something that suddenly emerges during adolescence. The CSBI was developed not only to establish this baseline of normative sexual behaviors, but to evaluate children when sexual abuse is suspected. Data from this research with the CSBI, including large samples of children with no known history of sexual abuse, indicated that the most frequent sexual behaviors included self-stimulation, exhibitionism, and behaviors related to personal boundaries. The more "intrusive" behaviors (fondling, oral sex, anal penetration, and/or vaginal penetration) were clearly less often observed (Friedrich et al., 1998; see also Grant & Lundeberg, 2009).

Friedrich and colleagues, in their development and implementation of the CSBI, have pursued the most comprehensive examination of childhood sexual behaviors in the last two decades. The CSBI (Friedrich, 1997) is a 38-item protocol that asks parents to rate the frequency of observed sexual behaviors in their children, using a 4-point Likert scale (0, never; 1, less than once a month; 2, 1 to 3 times per month; 3, once a week or more) during the previous 6-month period. Designed for completion by parents of children ages 2–12, the CSBI captures parental or caregiver observations of a range of sexual behaviors. CSBI domains include boundary problems, exhibitionism, gender role behavior, self-stimulation, sexual anxiety, sexual interest, sexual intrusiveness, sexual knowledge, and voyeuristic behaviors (Grant & Lundeberg, 2009). Despite the obvious limitations as a parent report measure, particularly since the topic of sexuality and sexual behaviors creates a wide range of emotions in parents, the data derived from the CSBI can be extremely useful in determining the most appropriate treatment path for both a child and his or her family. Administering the CSBI periodically throughout treatment is also useful to monitor progress.

The research conducted by Friedrich and colleagues (1998) provides a guide to differentiate developmentally related sexual behaviors from behaviors that are frequently found in children who have been sexually abused. In general, normative data for the 2- to 5-year-old age group suggest that boys at this age often stand too close to people; touch their own private parts while in public; touch or try to touch their mothers' or other women's breasts; touch their own private parts when at home; and may try to look at people when they are nude or undressing. Normative data for the 6- to 9-year-old age group suggest that boys and girls at this age often touch their own private parts when at home, and try to look at people when they are nude or undressing. Normative data for the 10- to 12-year-old age group suggest that most boys and girls start to become very interested in the opposite sex during this time.

In Friedrich et al's. (1998) sample of 1,114 children ages 2–12 (who were screened for the absence of sexual abuse), sexual behavior was related to a child's age, maternal education, family sexuality, family stress, family violence, and hours per week in day care. The relative frequency of sexual behaviors within this age range was found to be similar to the findings of two earlier studies (Kendall-Tackett, Williams, & Finkelhor, 1993; Friedrich, Grambsch, Broughton, Kuiper, & Bielke, 1991).

These additional findings were as follows: 2-year-old children were found to be relatively sexual (compared with 10- to 12-year-olds), and children became increasingly sexual up to the age of 5 years. Another reduction in display of sexual behaviors was found to occur after age 9. However, 11-year-old girls showed a slight rise in sexual behavior (primarily stemming from this age group's increased interest in the opposite sex). At age 12, boys also showed a similar slight increase in display of sexual behaviors, again attributable to an increase in interest in the opposite sex during this period of their development.

Kellogg and the Committee on Child Abuse and Neglect (2009) have concurred with Friedrich et al. (1991, 1998) that problematic sexual behavior is also significantly related to both family violence and total life stress. This group notes that

> both of these [factors] have been shown to be related to behavior problems in children, and to the extent that sexual behavior can be problematic, it is likely that a similar connection exists. Life stress may reflect less consistent parenting and as a result may predispose a child to act out in a variety of ways. Family violence is a model for boundary problems and intrusive behavior range from normal and developmentally appropriate to abusive and violent. While earlier studies have suggested a strong correlation between sexual abuse and sexual behavior problems in children, more recent studies have broadened this perspective, recognizing a number of additional stressors, family characteristics, and environmental factors that are associated with intrusive and frequent sexual behaviors. Clinicians must first distinguish age-appropriate and normal sexual behaviors from behaviors that are developmentally inappropriate and/or abusive. (p. 992)

Specific Normative Sexual Behaviors

Infants and preschool-age children (age 4 or younger) are naturally disinhibited or immodest and may openly display curiosity about bodies and bodily functions (Hagan, Shaw, & Duncan, 2008; American Academy of Pediatrics, 2005). As summarized by Gil (1993), "It is common for children in this age group to 'discover' that when certain parts of the body are touched, poked, rubbed, or otherwise stimulated, pleasant sensations occur. When something pleasurable occurs, children may seek to repeat the event; the younger the child the more likely the repetition occurs by accident" (p. 22). Specifically, common or age-typical sexual behaviors in preschool-age children include rubbing private parts; exploring and touching private parts (in public and private); showing private parts to others; trying to touch their mothers' or other women's breasts; removing clothes/wanting to be nude; voyeuristic behaviors (attempting to see other people nude or undressing); asking questions about bodies and bodily functions; and/or talking to children their own age about bodily functions (Hagan et al., 2008).

According to the American Academy of Pediatrics (2005), common or age-typical sexual behaviors in young children (approximately 4–6 years of age) include masturbation, or purposeful touching of private parts (occasionally in the presence of others); voyeuristic behaviors; mimicking of adult sexual behaviors (e.g., kissing, dating rituals, or holding hands); talking about private parts; exploring private parts with children their own age (e.g., playing "doctor").

The American Academy of Pediatrics (2005) describes the following common or age-typical sexual behaviors in school-age children (approximately 7–12 years old): masturbation (usually in private); playing games with children their own age that involve sexual behavior (e.g., "boyfriend/girlfriend," "truth or dare"); voyeuristic behaviors; looking at pictures of naked or partially naked people; viewing/listening to sexual content in various media (television, movies, games, the Internet, music, etc.); increasingly preferring more privacy and more reluctant to talk to adults about sexual concerns; and becoming increasingly sexually attracted to peers. School-age children are becoming aware of social and family rules, so they become more modest and prefer more privacy than they did prior to age 7. Masturbation and sexual play does continue, but children are more likely to hide this activity from adults. They begin to seek out, and become increasingly interested in, sexual content in the media. Exchanging what they learn with peers and telling jokes about sex are common for this age group. This age (if not earlier) is the time to start providing children with accurate information and give them opportunities to question, explore, and evaluate their own and their families' and cultures' attitudes toward sexuality and sexual behaviors. Family, friendship, and other relationships are core components of healthy sexuality at this stage of children's psychosexual development (American Academy of Pediatrics, 2005).

In general, "typical" childhood sexual play and exploration occur between children who play together regularly and know each other well;

occur between children of the same general age and physical size; are spontaneous and unplanned; are infrequent; are voluntary (none of the involved children seem uncomfortable or upset); and are easily diverted when parents tell them to stop and explain privacy rules (Gil, 1993; Friedrich, 2007; Hagan et al., 2008). Gil (1993) describes differences between typical and atypical sexual play as follows:

> The dynamics of age-appropriate, exploratory sex play between young children usually includes spontaneity, joy, laughter, embarrassment, and sporadic levels of inhibition and disinhibition. On the other hand, problem sexual behaviors have themes of dominance, coercion, threats, and force. Children seem agitated, anxious, fearful, or intense. They have higher levels of arousal, and the sexual activity may be habitual. It is as though no other activity gives the same degree of pleasure, excitement, comfort, or reassurance, and it becomes the focus of the child's life. This behavior is usually unresponsive to any parental or caregiver limits or distractions. (p. 32)

Clinicians are therefore encouraged to consider the following criteria when presented with situations of children engaging in questionable sexual behaviors with other children: (1) age difference between the children; (2) size difference; (3) status difference (relative equality, such as that between siblings who are close in age, or inequality, such as a "larger bully vs. smaller victim" dynamic); and (4) other dynamics (e.g., factors leading up to the behavior, each child's contribution to the behavior, the tone of the interaction).

Silovsky and Bonner (2004) summarize ideas articulated by leading professionals in this narrow field of study (some of which overlap with points made above) that should be taken into consideration in distinguishing normative sexual play from sexual behavior problems. Normative sexual play is usually exploratory and spontaneous; occurs by mutual agreement; typically involves children of similar size, age, or developmental level; does not evoke high levels of arousal, anger, or anxiety; decreases or stops when appropriately redirected by caregivers; and can be controlled by increased monitoring. When the sexual interactions become problematic, the behavior is frequent or repeated despite appropriate caregiver redirection; occurs often and interferes with other activities; occurs between children of different ages, sizes, and/or developmental levels; is aggressive or forced; does not decrease or stop when appropriately redirected; and/or causes harm to the child or others. In other words, the behavior ceases to reflect normative curiosity and play between children, and takes on qualities that leave one or both children feeling anxious, confused, or frightened.

PROBLEMATIC SEXUAL BEHAVIORS

Recognizing, understanding, and responding to children with sexual behavior problems constitute an emerging area of research and practice. The robust data that have emerged in the past two decades seem to challenge early assumptions about such children (Silovsky & Bonner, 2003a). We have already provided some definitions of childhood sexual behavior problems in Chapter One. In addition, Silovsky and Bonner (2003a) define children with sexual behavior problems as "children 12 years and under who demonstrate developmentally inappropriate or aggressive sexual behavior. This definition includes self-focused sexual behavior, such as excessive masturbation, and aggressive sexual behavior towards others that may include coercion or force" (p. 1). These authors provide six further qualifiers before a behavior should be considered problematic: It (1) occurs at a high frequency; (2) interferes with the child's social or cognitive development; (3) occurs with coercion, intimidation, or force; (4) is associated with emotional distress; (5) occurs between children of significantly different ages and/or developmental abilities; and/or (6) repeatedly occurs in secrecy after intervention by caregivers. According to Friedrich (2007), this definition is an excellent starting point; however, the application of the definition still relies on the adults in a child's life. It is also important to note that children of the same age are capable of engaging in hurtful sexual behavior problems, so relying on the single criterion of age/developmental difference is insufficient.

Terminology and Assessment Issues

The term "sexual behavior problems" describes a spectrum of problematic behaviors in children, from overly sexualized behaviors (e.g., excessive or public masturbation) to behaviors that are intrusive, aggressive, and/or harmful to others. Defining the first two of these latter terms may be helpful. "Intrusive" sexual behaviors are behaviors that involve others, including animals, other children, or adults. "Aggressive" sexual behaviors include behaviors that (1) persist after limits are set; (2) involve planning how to touch other children sexually; (3) include one child's forcing others to engage in sex acts; and (4) include acts of physical penetration, such as inserting a finger or objects into another child's vagina or rectum (Friedrich, 2007). The nature of a particular child's sexual behavior problem must be established at the outset through careful assessment, as we discuss in detail in Chapter Four of this book.

When children are referred to mental health professionals because of concerns about possible sexual behavior problems, Silovsky et al. (2012) assert that the first clinical task is to do a comprehensive assessment that gathers information on the type, frequency, duration, severity, and history of the problem. In addition, it is important to note how the problems have been addressed to date, and what children's responsiveness has been to adult interventions. The social and cultural context of the sexual behaviors is also relevant. In their comprehensive review of the research, Silovsky et al. (2012) discuss common co-occurring clinical concerns clinicians need to assess. These include (1) trauma-related symptoms for children who have experienced trauma; (2) other internalizing symptoms; (3) disruptive behavior disorder symptoms (e.g., symptoms of ADHD or oppositional defiant disorder); (4) social skills deficits; and (5) learning problems (p. 404). Finally, many parents or caregivers may see any childhood sexual behaviors as problematic or sufficient reason for concern. In particular, for many parents/caregivers, any sexual behaviors in their children may elicit fears that the children have been sexually abused (and/or may grow up to be abusers), and these fears can be conveyed to the children. Because such fears can be so strong and can have such serious effects, we discuss abuse-reactive behaviors next.

Sexually Reactive or Abuse-Reactive Behaviors

Friedrich and colleagues' research and CSBI data indicate that children who have been sexually abused tend to insert objects into their vaginal or anal openings more than nonabused children do (Friedrich et al., 1991; Friedrich, 2007). However, this does not imply that nonabused children never engage in this behavior. The behavior itself cannot be interpreted in isolation; nor should parents conclude that abuse has occurred (or ask questions about possible abuse) before the child has undergone a developmentally sensitive assessment. According to Gil (1993), "many children who have been overstimulated sexually cannot integrate these experiences in a meaningful way. This can result in children acting out the confusion in the form of more advanced or frequent sexual behaviors, heightened interest and/or knowledge beyond what would be expected of that age" (p. 45).

As Gil (1993) reminds us, it is also possible that a child who makes excessive contact with his or her genitals can be indicating a medical problem. In addition, sometimes children who masturbate with dirty fingers can inadvertently cause a urinary tract infection, which may cause them to touch or squirm in order to relieve the pain.

Chaffin et al. (2006) and Friedrich (2007) concur that rates of sexual behavior problems are higher in clinically referred children who have been sexually abused than in children without abuse histories. Preschool children who have been sexually abused are at particular risk, with about a third demonstrating some sexual behavior problems. These problems occur less frequently as an issue for school-age children who have been sexually abused, with only about 6% of such children demonstrating sexual behavior problems (Kendall-Tackett, Williams, & Finkelhor, 1993).

Children who have been sexually abused can act out sexually for a variety of reasons, but more often than not they are probably trying to deal with their own sexual abuse, sometimes by acting out the more active role of victimizer versus the passive role of victim. However, this behavior can occur out of children's conscious awareness, sometimes when something has triggered an intrusive thought or feeling that they cannot tolerate. The question of why some child victims abuse others and many others do not is an important subject for research. Gil (1993) goes on to say:

> Sexually reactive children often feel deep shame, intense guilt, and pervasive anxiety about sexuality. Often the sexual behaviors of abuse reactive children are limited to their own bodies—that is, masturbation, exposing or inserting objects in themselves, etc. If they do engage in sexual behaviors with other children, the difference in age is usually not great, and they typically do not force other children into sexual behaviors. (p. 45)

Sexual Aggression and Other Severe Behavior Problems

In Chapter One, we have cited Chaffin et al.'s (2006) observation that "the most concerning [sexual behavior problem] cases involve substantial age or developmental inequalities; more advanced sexual behaviors; aggression, force or coercion; and harm or the potential for harm" (pp. 3–4). Nevertheless, as suggested by Friedrich (2007), everyone who works in this field needs to appreciate the tremendous developmental differences that exist among children with even such severe sexual behavior problems as these, adolescent sexual offenders, and adult sexual offenders. The therapy and other interventions provided for each of these groups must reflect a thorough understanding of these developmental differences.

Child welfare systems struggle with how to manage children with severe sexual behavior problems in foster care (Farmer & Pollock, 1998). When a higher-risk child is placed in a foster home, and sexual contact occurs between this child and another child in the home, the foster placement can be disrupted; the child with sexual behavior problems is typically moved to a setting where no other children are present.

> Some foster children can be so sexually focused that their best hope is to be placed either in a residential facility or with a female foster parent so that no adult male is accused of sexual abuse. These children then may lose contact with siblings whom they were placed with initially. Their adoptability, in those cases when that is an option, is also reduced. (Friedrich, 2007, p. 11)

Such severe problems occur in only a small minority of cases, however. Current data (primarily from the research conducted by Friedrich and colleagues) give clinicians the opportunity to educate not only parents, but also the professionals who become involved and who may also assume that sexual abuse is the underlying reason for all sexual behavior problems. Research has concluded that a broad range of sexual behaviors is exhibited by children for whom there is no reason to suspect sexual abuse (Friedrich et al., 1991, 1998; Friedrich, 2007). Again, a thorough, developmentally appropriate assessment is best to determine what may be driving these problem behaviors for individual children.

Children with sexual behavior problems are quite diverse, as emphasized in Chapter One, and no *profile* for such children exists to date. That is, no clear pattern of demographic, psychological, or social factors distinguishes children with sexual behavior problems from other groups of children (Chaffin et al., 2002). Contributing factors may include child maltreatment, coercive or neglectful parenting practices, exposure to sexually explicit media, living in a highly sexualized environment, and exposure to family violence, as well as individual factors and heredity (Chaffin et al., 2006; Friedrich et al., 2001; Langstrom, Grann, & Lichtenstein, 2002; Merrick, Litrownik, Everson, & Cox, 2008). "Sexual behavior problems . . . do not represent a medical/psychological syndrome or a specific diagnosable disorder" (Chaffin et al., 2006, p. 3); rather, these are behaviors that society considers unacceptable, that can be hurtful to others, and that cause impairment in functioning.

SUMMARY

Concerns have grown and persist about what constitute normative versus problematic sexual behaviors. It is therefore important for a mental health professional to undertake a purposeful and comprehensive assessment of each child to determine the type and consistency of specific sexual behaviors, the child's responsiveness to limits, and risk factors to other children (and animals). There appears to be a continuum of challenging behaviors that can emerge in children for a variety of reasons; a great deal of research has attempted to clarify the nature of these behaviors and their possible causes. It becomes important to determine whether a child's behavior can be addressed by coaching parents/other caregivers to respond with empathy and firm limits, or whether the child and family will require mental health services targeting the reduction of sexual behavior problems. Once an adequate assessment has taken place, some treatment approaches have been shown to be necessary and helpful, and these are discussed in Chapters Five and Six.

CHAPTER THREE

The Climate of Childhood Sexualization

Michael, a 10-year-old boy, was referred for an assessment after a school suspension for repeatedly using inappropriate language about sexual acts, making sexualized gestures, and (in the most recent incident) soliciting a female peer to touch his penis on the playground. Michael told the young girl that if she told anyone about what he was doing, he would tell everyone that she had approached him and asked whether she could touch his penis. She refused his advances and told her parents a few weeks later, after he started bullying her on the playground.

Michael was the only child of a single mother who worked two jobs. He attended an after-school program for 3 hours each weekday, and he spent every other weekend with his father. There was little to no communication between the parents regarding most matters, including rules about or limits on Michael's access to electronic and other media. Michael had recently received a cell phone with Internet access from his father, reportedly so that he could call his father when he needed or wanted to. Michael's mother had opposed giving a 10-year-old a cell phone, but to no avail—and, because it was in the father's name, she had no way to monitor Michael's calls, texts, or Internet history. Computer access at his mother's house was reported by the mother as "limited but with parental controls." During the intake interview with his mother, she admitted that she had limited knowledge about computers and Internet safety, and did not know how to check to see what sites Michael was visiting. During the intake interview with Michael's father, the father stated that he did not apply parental controls because "I trust my son and he'd tell me if he wanted more information," and "Boys will find a way to learn about sex, regardless of computer settings . . . pornography was around long before the Internet."

During the assessment, Michael himself reported that he had been exposed to sexual content and sexual images in the following ways. A fifth-grade boy in his after-school program had brought in images he printed from a pornographic website, and had shared these with Michael and two other children. The images included oral sex acts, bondage ("a woman in a dog collar tied to a bed"), and two men "having sex with each other in the butt." Michael had then typed the following keywords into his father's home computer: "penis in mouth," "girl tied up," and "men having sex." He had continued similar Internet searches on his father's computer every other weekend for 3 months prior to the assessment, and had been sharing images with the boy who originally introduced him to pornography. They now "shared pictures" after school (in the after-school program, the staff-to-student ratio was 25:1).

Michael admitted that he had found ways to access similar sites on his mother's computer, adding that "she never checks anyway." When asked about the parental control settings on the home computer, he responded, "Well, they do work. I reset it with a password, so now my mom is locked out." When asked how often he looked at pictures about sex, Michael responded, "Whenever I want . . . I got a phone with Internet for my birthday." When asked how often he thought about the images he saw, he responded, "When I'm bored." When asked whether he had talked to his father about what images he has seen, or asked either parent any questions about sex, Michael responded, "No, it's too embarrassing, and then they could just take away my phone and computer."

Gabby, a 7-year-old girl, was referred for therapy by her parents following an incident in which Gabby invited a same-age male peer to her bedroom and was found with her pants down, sitting close to the boy on her bed. The boy told Gabby's mother he had told Gabby he didn't want to play the "girl–boy game" and wanted to go home. Gabby's mother reported that she remembered Gabby's friend had looked upset when he asked to go home and had since refused to play with Gabby. In addition to the referring incident, several sexualized behaviors were reported.

Gabby was the youngest of six children (there were four teenagers in the household). There was no reported history of abuse or neglect. Given her age, if such an incident was isolated and did not create distress for either child, I (J. A. S.) would probably focus on brief parent coaching rather than therapy for the child and/or family. However, following the parent intake and completion of the CSBI (Friedrich, 1997), on which Gabby obtained elevated scores as compared to same-age female peers, I recommended brief therapy for the child with periodic parent–child sessions.

Gabby's parents had begun to worry about her excessive interest in the opposite sex and the fact that she seemed to know much more about sex than her peers. The parents said that they had prepared themselves for these concerns when Gabby was older, but they felt she was too young to be asking boys to be her boyfriends, bragging about the number of "boyfriends" she had, and trying to kiss her brothers and father on the lips. When she wanted to kiss open-mouthed, she referred to wanting to kiss "like they do on TV," and it had become difficult to keep her from watching TV shows that were inappropriate for her age. Several times after the parents thought Gabby was asleep, they would find her watching adult programming late at night. She protested that "cartoons are for babies." Her mother also noted that shopping had become a power struggle, because Gabby wanted her mother to buy her more "sexy clothes" and accused the mother of wanting to baby her. During the intake, it also became apparent that the parents had different views about Gabby's behavior. For example, at one point when her mother was talking about clothes-shopping difficulties, her father laughed, stating, "She's all girl." The mother added, "See . . . her father encourages her," at which point he became defensive and withdrawn.

Gabby came to her first assessment session wearing a tight-fitting t-shirt and very short shorts with "Princess" embroidered across the backside. She seemed to prance around the waiting room, trying to get the attention of several teenage boys who were waiting for their appointments.

The themes in Gabby's play centered almost entirely around romantic relationships and engaging in activities (games) that would be more appropriate for adolescents. She told a story about school that was focused on boys in her class and on girls' not liking her because "they are jealous of my boyfriends." Gabby's primary activities at home centered around fashion, makeup, and "doing hair." She stated that she couldn't wait to be 8 years old, because that was how old her parents told her she had to be to start wearing "shimmering lip gloss." When asked about her favorite television shows, Gabby described shows from the Disney Channel in which the characters were all teenagers.

My immediate concerns about this child were the mixed messages she was getting from her parents, her access to unsupervised TV (a set was in her room), and other stimulating environmental factors that might be involved (especially given her teenage siblings). My task was to determine where this apparent overattention to sexuality was coming from, and what (if anything) could be done to help her regulate what seemed an excessive interest in sex, particularly as reflected in her more recent acting-out behaviors with other children.

*   *   *

Exposure to sexually explicit media and living in a highly sexualized environment are factors that can contribute to sexual behavior problems in childhood (Chaffin et al., 2006; Friedrich et al., 2003). Containing a child's world to developmentally appropriate material about sexuality and sexual acts is becoming increasingly difficult for all parents/caregivers, and controlling for these external factors is increasingly challenging for mental health professionals tasked with assisting families of children with sexual behavior problems.

Among the most critical aspects of work with children who have developed sexual behavior problems are addressing and focusing on safety issues and supervisory needs. First, addressing a child's access to various media and the extent to which the child may live in a sexualized environment requires immediate attention in the form of education for the caregivers. As suggested by the title of Levin and Kilbourne's (2008) book, *So Sexy So Soon*, the issue is not that children are learning about sex. The issues are what they are learning, the age at which they are learning it, and who is teaching them. "Many children live in a world that we expect to be contained and protective. But even the most protected children are exposed to sexual material that can be confusing, exciting, and overstimulating" (Lamb, 2006, p. 5).

The home environment, including the extent to which that environment "blocks" messages from televisions, movies, and the Internet, is of primary importance in the sexual socialization of children. For many contemporary children, a constant flow of unfiltered information is coming into their daily lives via portable multimedia devices. These devices, which may be provided even to very young children, often have wireless capability no longer limited to what is immediately available in most homes. Children can be flooded with messages and images without their parents' or other caregivers' awareness—that is, without an opportunity for adults to screen or clarify what children see, to set necessary limits, and to help the children process complex messages.

Uncontrolled and unfiltered messages about sex and sexuality can be overwhelming, overstimulating, and confusing for young and school-age children, and parents are finding it harder and harder to learn what their children are exposed to outside the confines of a protective home. Concerns are no longer limited to what might be found in another child's home, but what material, images, or language might have been found on a peer's laptop, phone, or portable device with wireless access. As stated by Levin and Kilbourne (2008),

> Today there is grave disconnection between the values caring parents want to convey to their children about relationships, sex, and sexuality and the messages conveyed by the popular culture. Many parents feel they need to fight the current cultural messages at every turn with younger and younger children. (p. 162)

WHERE WE ARE WITH MARKETING TO CHILDREN

Children are growing up in an increasingly sophisticated marketing environment that influences their thoughts, perceptions, preferences, and behaviors. Images of sex and sexuality are everywhere. Advertisements are explicitly erotic, and music videos are almost invariably full of sexual themes and suggestive lyrics. American marketing and advertising support the economy by promoting the sale of goods and services to consumers, and young children are a new target group and therefore increasingly attentive to marketing strategies. As suggested by Sandra Calvert (2008), marketers have targeted children for decades, but two recent trends have contributed to the increased interest in children: (1) the discretionary income of children and their power to influence their parents purchases have increased over time, and (2) there has been a tremendous increase in the amount of available media space just for children and children's products. Levin and Kilbourne (2008) offer a detailed historical perspective on the upward trend toward marketing to children from the 1970s to the present day.

These rapid shifts and trends in media and children's usage have not occurred in tandem with a clear understanding of the ways in which children's development may be impacted. Young children cannot discern the full subliminal messages of advertisements, and school-age or older children cannot always comprehend the intent of newer marketing strategies that blur the line between program content and commercial advertising. As suggested by Calvert (2008), television remains the primary venue for advertising; however, new approaches to reaching the child consumer through online media and wireless devices are constantly being explored. In what M. Gigi Durham (2008) calls a global phenomenon, on an average day with more and more accessibility in the average U.S. household, children can be bombarded with a media environment that includes over 200 cable television networks, over 5,000 magazine titles, 10,500 radio stations, in excess of 30 million websites, and 122,000 newly published books. According to Durham, in *The Lolita Effect,* the turn of the century, or the new millennium, "has spawned an intriguing phenomenon: the sexy little girl" (p. 24).

In 1978, a Federal Trade Commission (FTC) report concluded that children under the age of 7 are not cognitively able to evaluate even child-oriented television advertising (a conclusion that the American Psychological Association (APA) later confirmed; see Wilcox et al., 2004). The U.S. Congress sought to empower the FTC to design greater regulatory efforts, but opposition from the powerful entertainment and marketing industries prevented regulations in children's advertising from being enacted.

Anyone who has even the slightest interest in marketing patterns in children's advertising has noticed a persistent and bold tendency toward the sexualization of younger and younger children. It is very clear that advertisers have identified children as consumers and have created daring strategies to gain their attention. A parent of a six-year-old told me the following: "I used to let my daughter watch the Disney channel because she loved it so much; one day, after having her constantly request a certain product, I took a focused look at the advertising. I was shocked at how blatantly they were introducing older children who looked very sexy and grown up to sell their products. From that day on, I only let her watch TV if she left the room when the commercials came on."

Another trend rampant throughout printed ads is the subtle and direct merging of sex and violence that has influenced the development of much more gender-stereotyped advertising. Different programs, and products linked with them, were developed specifically for either boys or girls. Initially, girls' programming focused on sweet behavior and pretty appearance, with shows like Care Bears, My Little Pony, and, most recently, Princess Sophia. But gradually and consistently, increasingly explicit sexual imagery is used; sexiness and mean-spirited behavior have crept into shows like the Powerpuff Girls and toys like the Bratz dolls. A recent MTV Awards show stirred up quite a controversy when former child-star Miley Cyrus danced in a blatantly sexually-provocative way dressed in a very skimpy outfit. Unfortunately, the controversy might have been precisely the kind of attention that marketers desire since this dance was the event that gleaned the greatest media attention. Just as sex and a sexy physical appearance became the primary themes in the programming for girls, aggression and violence became common themes in the programming for boys, with such highly successful shows (and related toys) as Masters of the Universe, Transformers, Mighty Morphin Power Rangers, and the Avengers. These trends are sometimes criticized or challenged, which briefly draws more attention to them, but nonetheless continue to be daily features of our society that are increasingly influential on the minds of young children in ways that we cannot yet fully appreciate.

Because entertainers whose target audience is children or young teens are also "selling" a "commodity" of sorts, the extent to which it has become commonplace to describe young singers as "hot!" is likewise a concern. Stars like Rihanna, Lady Gaga, and Nicki Minaj wear very sexy clothing and dance provocatively while singing songs with very sexual and sometimes violent lyrics. These performers are presented for young girls to view as role models—and for young boys to see as desirable.

THE SCOPE OF THE MEDIA CHALLENGE: HOW OFTEN ARE CHILDREN GETTING THESE MESSAGES?

A report published by the Henry J. Kaiser Family Foundation (KFF) found that many children spent more time involved with media than on anything else but sleeping (Kunkel et al., 2005). The KFF has conducted a series of studies and compiled several reports over the last decade that document the growing challenge posed by the mass media's influence on children's lives. An earlier report from KFF, Zero to Six: Electronic Media in the Lives of Infants, Toddlers and Preschoolers (Rideout, Vandewater, & Wartella, 2003), found that 36% of children under the age of 6 lived in households where a television was turned on "always" or "most of the time." Thirty percent of infants (birth to age 3) and 43% of young children (4–6 years) had a television in their bedrooms. These rates suggest that even infants and toddlers are watching television or movies without a caregiver present, and that television is an essential feature in the home environment from the very beginning of children's lives.

Moreover, the KFF's Zero to Six report (Rideout et al., 2003) found that nearly three out of four young children (73%) had a computer at home, and that 49% had a video game player. In some ways, new media were already trumping old: Almost twice as many children lived in a home with Internet access (63%) as with a newspaper subscription (34%). Nearly all of them (97%) had products (clothes, toys, etc.) based on characters from TV shows or movies. Although unsurprisingly high percentages of children (89% or more) in the 0–6 age group had listened to music, had read or been read to, had watched TV, and had watched videos or DVDs, more unexpected findings were that nearly half (48%) of all these children had used a computer and that 30% had played video games. According to their parents, these young children spent an average of about 2 hours a day with screen media (1:58)—about the same amount of time that they spent playing outside (2:01), and far more time than they spent reading or being read to (39 minutes).

The 2005 KFF report (Kunkel et al., 2005) included data from a survey of the screen habits of children ages 8–18 years. On average, these youngsters were exposed to 8½ hours of media content each day—an increase of over an hour a day from 5 years earlier. It also reported that approximately two-thirds of this age group had a television in their bedrooms, and that about half also had a video game player attached to or in addition to the television.

According to Rideout et al. (2003), these rapid increases in children's use of various media have not been accompanied by similar expansion in our knowledge of how these media may affect children's social, emotional, cognitive, or physical development. These issues are of great concern not only to parents, but to educators, health care providers, policy makers, and advocates. Early childhood experts argue that it is especially important to understand young children's media use, because development is so rapid and so vulnerable at at the youngest ages.

Regarding gender differences in the use of media, Rideout et al. (2003) found that at younger ages boys and girls seemed to spend about the same amounts of time using various media, to develop the same basic media use skills, and to do so at about the same ages. By the ages of 4–6, however, boys were more likely to play video games and to play for longer periods of time. This contributed to an 18-minute difference between boys and girls of these ages in the average amount of time they spent in front of screen media each day. Another gender difference was found in the percentage of boys versus girls who had imitated aggressive behaviors they saw on TV (45% of boys, compared to 28% of girls). This difference was especially striking among the 4- to 6-year-olds (59% of boys vs. 35% of girls). It remained unclear, however, whether boys were actually watching shows with more violent content, or whether they were simply more likely to copy the violent behaviors they saw.

The 2003 KFF study thus documented the immersion of the very youngest children in the world of electronic and interactive media. As Rideout et al. (2003) noted, the effects of this level of exposure on children's development remain unknown, but the issue plainly demands immediate attention from primary caregivers, educators, researchers, and health care professionals.

George Gerbner, professor of communications and dean emeritus of the Annenberg School of Communication in Philadelphia, has directed a number of studies of mass communications and its effects on culture. Although Gerbner (1994) stated the following in regard to television, it can be said of the newer media as well:

> The alienating culture of television has taken the place of other forms of communication that at one time tied us together in families and communities, and gave us all the opportunity to participate in creating and passing along our cultural story. For the first time in human history, children are hearing most of the stories, most of the time, not from their parents or school or churches or neighbors, but from a handful of global conglomerates that have something to sell. It is impossible to overestimate the radical effect that this has on the way our children grow up, the way we live, and the way we conduct our affairs.

SEXUALIZATION OF GIRLS

The discussion in this section is adapted from the Executive Summary of the Report of the APA Task Force on the Sexualization of Girls (2007).* According to the APA Task Force, nearly every media form that has been studied provides overwhelming evidence for the "sexualization of women, including television, music videos, music lyrics, movies, magazines, sports media, video games, the Internet, and advertising." The Task Force defines "sexualization" as occurring when (1) "a person's

---

* Copyright 2007 by the American Psychological Association. Adapted with permission. The official citation that should be used in referencing this material is American Psychological Association (APA) Task Force on the Sexualization of Girls (2007). Executive summary. No further reproduction or distribution is permitted without written permission from the American Psychological Association.

value comes only from his or her sexual appeal or behavior, to the exclusion of other characteristics;" (2) "a person is held to a standard that equates physical attractiveness (narrowly defined) with being sexy;" (3) "a person is sexually objectified—that is, made into a thing for others' sexual use, rather than seen as a person with the capacity for independent action and decision making;" and/or (4) "sexuality is inappropriately imposed upon a person." Any one of these four conditions is an indication of sexualization. The fourth condition (the inappropriate imposition of sexuality) is particularly applicable to children, since "when children are imbued with adult sexuality, it is often imposed upon them rather than chosen by them."

Some studies have examined forms of media that are especially popular with children and adolescents, such as video games and teen-focused magazines. In study after study, findings have indicated that women are portrayed more often than men in a sexual manner, and are objectified as defined above more often. Moreover, a narrow, unrealistic image of physical beauty is heavily emphasized as the model of femininity for young girls to strive for.

Other studies focused on the sexualization of female characters across all ages, but most focused specifically on young adult women. Although few studies examined the prevalence of sexualized portrayals of girls in particular, these few have found that such sexualization may be becoming common. For example, O'Donohue, Gold, and McKay (1997) coded advertisements over a 40-year period in five magazines targeted to men, women, or a general adult readership. Although relatively few (1.5%) of the ads portrayed children in a sexualized manner, of those that did, 85% depicted girls rather than boys. Furthermore, the percentage of sexualizing ads increased over time.

Although extensive analyses documenting the sexualization of girls in particular had not yet been conducted when the APA Task Force (2007) published its report, individual examples can easily be found. These include advertisements, dolls and other toys, clothing, and television programs of the types described by Levin and Kilbourne (2008) and described earlier in this chapter

The Task Force has noted that parents may contribute to their daughters' sexualization in a number of ways. For example, parents may convey the message that an attractive physical appearance is the most important goal for girls. Some may even permit or encourage their daughters to obtain plastic surgery to help meet that goal. Peers of both genders have also been found to contribute to girls' sexualization—other girls by exerting pressure to conform to standards of thinness and sexiness (Eder, 1995; Nichter, 2000), and boys by objectifying and harassing girls. Finally, parents, teachers, and peers, as well as others (e.g., other relatives, coaches, or strangers), may sexually abuse, assault, or otherwise criminally exploit girls—the most destructive types of sexualization.

If girls buy (or ask their parents to buy for them) clothes and other products intended to make them look sexy, and if they pattern their identities after the "hot" celebrities they admire, they are actually sexualizing themselves. Girls also do this when they think of themselves in objectified terms. Researchers have identified "self-objectification" as a process in which girls come to think of and treat their own bodies as objects of other persons' desires (Fredrickson & Roberts, 1997; McKinley & Hyde, 1996). Many studies have documented that self-objectification is found more often in women than in men, and it is not surprising that young girls have suffered greatly to maintain their perceived standards of beauty.

In the cognitive domain, self-objectification has been repeatedly shown to decrease concentration and focused attention, and thus to impair performance on mental activities such as mathematical computations or logical reasoning (Frederickson, Roberts, Noll, Quinn, & Twenge, 1998; Gapinski, Brownell, & LaFrance, 2003; Hebl, King, & Lin, 2004). For example, Fredrickson et al. (1998) studied college students who were asked to try on and evaluate either a swimsuit or a sweater while they were alone in a dressing room. As they waited for 10 minutes wearing the garment, they completed a math test. The results revealed that young women in swimsuits did significantly worse on the math problems than did those wearing sweaters; no differences were found for young men.

In the emotional domain, sexualization and objectification decrease confidence in and comfort with one's own body; this can lead to a variety of negative emotional consequences, such as shame, anxiety, and even self-disgust. An association between self-objectification on the one hand, and appearance-related anxiety and feelings of shame on the other, has been found in 12- to 13-year-old girls (Slater & Tiggemann, 2002) as well as in adult women.

Other research has connected sexualization to three common mental health problems among girls and women: eating disorders, low self-esteem, and depression or depressed mood (Abramson & Valene, 1991; Durkin & Paxton, 2002; Harrison, 2000; Hofschire & Greenberg, 2002; Mills, Polivy, Herman, & Tiggemann, 2002; Stice, Schupak-Neuberg, Shaw, & Stein, 1994; Thomsen, Weber, & Brown, 2002; Ward, 2004).

Studies of both teenage girls and adult women have associated exposure to narrow representations of female beauty (e.g., the "thin ideal") with disordered eating attitudes and symptoms. Research also links exposure to sexualized female ideals with lower self-esteem, negative mood, and depressive symptoms among adolescent girls and women. In addition to the mental health consequences of sexualization, research suggests possible indirect effects on girls' and women's physical health.

Although sexual well-being is an important part of healthy development and overall well-being, evidence suggests that the sexualization of girls has negative effects on their development of healthy sexuality. Self-objectification has been linked directly to such sexual health indicators as decreased condom use and diminished sexual assertiveness among adolescent girls (Impett, Schooler, & Tolman, 2006).

Frequent exposure to narrow standards of attractiveness is also associated with unrealistic and/or negative expectations about sexuality. Shame and other negative effects that emerge during adolescence may lead to sexual problems in adulthood (Brotto, Heiman, & Tolman, 2009). Frequent exposures to media images that sexualize girls and women affect girls' concepts of femininity and sexuality. Girls and young women who more frequently consume or engage with mass media content more strongly endorse stereotypical depictions of women as sexual objects (Ward, 2002; Ward & Rivadeneyra, 1999; Zurbriggen & Morgan, 2006). They also judge appearance and physical attractiveness to be the primary basis of women's value.

THE SPECIAL PROBLEM OF PORNOGRAPHY

As our discussion to this point has made clear, children are increasingly confronted by overstimulating or sexualized material—up to and including "soft" and "hard-core" pornography—on their own or their parents' televisions and computers, at the homes of other children, or on multimedia devices that are increasingly shared among peers before and after school. Pornography poses a special problem: When young and school-age children view pornography, they are exposed to content that is well beyond their ability to comprehend. Pornographic images and messages, therefore, constitute an issue of emotional health: "Pornography objectifies people (especially women) and takes sex out of the context of even the pretense of a caring relationship. It is difficult for children to unlearn these attitudes" (Levin & Kilbourne, 2008, p. 47).

According to Levin and Kilbourne (2008), one survey showed that about 40% of children ages 10–17 had seen Internet pornography in the past year. Sixty-six percent of those children said that they did not want to view the images and had not sought them out; this suggests that they may have come upon the sexually explicit websites while searching the Internet for nonsexual information. An example of such a situation is offered by Sharon Lamb (2006): "God forbid your daughter wants to be a cheerleader and looks up cheerleading on the Web. She'll have to wade through 10 porn sites before she reaches a 'cheer club' " (p. 6).

Children today will inevitably be exposed to sexually explicit material, including pornography, and they need adults to help them understand it and process it (Lamb, 2006). Otherwise, they may be unable to deal with the resulting overstimulation. As Lamb describes it,

> the feeling of overstimulation is like being overwhelmed, maybe even excited, but not in a good way. Perhaps for some children or adolescents who seek out the state of overstimulation it feels good at first, but both the bodily and mental excitement are overwhelming, too much to manage, beyond one's resources, a stress. (p. 19)

WHAT CAN PARENTS/CAREGIVERS DO?

Providing Opportunities for Creative Play

As young children become more and more fanatical about playing with computers, watching TV, and entertaining themselves with video games, they miss out on opportunities for outdoor play or social interactions, both of which are often conducive to creative imagination. Some younger children find it "boring" to go for nature walks, for example, and the idea of doing quiet pretend play is unimaginable to them.

These days, unless parents and other caregivers create opportunities for children to play and interact with each other, their play may become stilted. Lamb (2006) states that "young children (ages 3 or 4) rarely engage in deeply complicated games of imagination with other children, but from age 5 onward, children's imaginative play with others can become intense and full of conflictual material" (p. 9). She goes on to say that in all children's play "there is mutual fun and there is bullying, there is friendship and there is exploitation, there is sharing and there is coercion. Children act out their interests as well as their worries in play and this more troublesome stuff does occur" (p. 10). However, when such play is supervised and kept within reasonable limits, it can be viewed as a safe forum where children's concerns are expressed through pretend situations, through role playing, and through storytelling. There are also times when children's earliest observations of sex and sexuality can be played out normatively—for example, when children playing innocently state, "You be the mommy and I'll be the daddy; let's play!"

Providing Modeling, Acceptance, and Guidance

Parents/caregivers play another critical role in terms of what they model, what they teach overtly and covertly, and how they respond to their children's behaviors and questions. Parental actions will influence when and where children express sexuality, and what to discuss with whom about sexuality. Children learn when sexual behaviors between people can begin by their parents' example. As children begin to experiment with nudity, touching, and exploring other's genitals, as well as with sexual games and sexual jokes, the guidelines set by parents and other caregivers teach them the appropriate balance for these activities in their lives. Exaggerated, angry, or horrified parental reactions (as well as parental ignoring due to discomfort or anxiety) send messages to children about themselves, sexuality, and sexual expression. If parents openly engage in relaxed, loving, consistent, appropriate modeling, "their actions provide a stronger message than their words" (Gil & Johnson, p. 15).

Among the most common parental concerns are children's masturbatory behaviors, and yet more and more parents are learning that this type of stimulation can be a part of normative development. In this area also, parental acceptance and guidance are pivotal to children's social development. "Children's genital awareness and self-touching, when accepted by parents, leads children to accept their bodies." (Gil & Johnson, p. 15).

For all children, it is important to recognize how sexual development is affected by their experience. For children with heightened sexual curiosity or preoccupation, or with actual sexual behavior problems, it is imperative. Parents are thus encouraged to discuss their thoughts and feelings about sexuality and develop a proactive plan in which scripts are developed, primary messages are clarified, and parents are not left feeling unprepared or caught off guard.

Most important is that parents understand that children learn by what they see, not just by what they are told, and that peer influence increases as they spend more time with friends at school and less time at home with their parents. In addition, children's interest in sexuality occurs gradually, not all at once, often without overt signs, as children begin to develop concepts of sex and sexuality from their parent's interactions, from their siblings and friends, and from television and printed media. Children will also have both internal and external pressures regarding gender conformity and gender identity, and these thoughts, feelings, and sensations can begin very early on.

Addressing "Sex Games" Appropriately and As Needed

Many children's early games about sexuality include an element of naïve and appropriate interest and curiosity. Some children's games can be coercive, as mentioned above. In such play children are usually working out conflicts, trying out appropriate responses, and using pretend play to express interest and curiosity. Minor and sporadic play using coercion can be part of children's play naturally, all over the world. These behaviors may be explored as children begin to determine what their values will be, how empathetic they are, and what the limits of acceptance might be from others. However, when this type of random play becomes a consistent pattern, when children's play seeps into their daily interactions with others, and/or when parents/caregivers are finding they cannot obtain empathic feelings from their children towards others, it may be useful to be cautious and address the problems directly.

There are many cases in which parents seek therapy due to their own discomfort with this topic, and mental health professionals can coach them to develop greater comfort by suggesting direct ways of approaching their concerns. There are other times when parents seek help after being worried for quite a while about their children's behaviors, and their concerns appear to be warranted. In these cases, mental health professionals will need to do comprehensive assessments, get to know the children, and find out what underlying concerns might be fueling the inappropriate behaviors.

WHAT ELSE CAN BE DONE TO COMBAT MEDIA INFLUENCES?

This chapter has made it clear that our mass media and popular culture, distributed in increasingly innovative ways to young children, are creating a generation of sexualized children. Fred Kaeser (2011) firmly states:

> A significant number of children are actually demonstrating sexual interest and/or sexual behavior at earlier ages than ever before in our society. Kids are being exposed to sexual matters that were previously only in the purview of adults and the greater the exposure the greater the consequences can be. When parents fail to counter and buffer the plethora of sexual stimuli that confront children, they are left to their own devices to manage what they experience. Unfortunately, many will be confused and have difficulty making sense of and putting into proper perspective what they are exposed to. Some will actually try to act out or mimic what they have been exposed to. Others, who may be developing a bullying persona, will begin to incorporate sexual behavior into their bullying behavior and engage in hurtful or intrusive sexual behavior towards other children. Frankly, I am alarmed over the number of five, six, seven, and eight year old children that molest other children. (I have NEVER received so many phone calls from school staff about this problem as I have the past ten to fifteen years.)

What other steps can be taken to deal with this situation, besides the ones recommended above for parents/caregivers? The APA Task Force (2007) has suggested that because the media are such important sources of sexualizing images, developing and implementing school-based media literacy training could be key in combating the influence of sexualization. There is an urgent need to teach critical skills for viewing various media, focusing specifically on the sexualization of women and girls. Other school-based approaches might include increasing girls' access to athletic and other extracurricular programs, as well as developing and implementing comprehensive sexuality education programs. Strategies that parents and other caregivers can pursue in regard to the media include learning about the impact of sexualization on girls and viewing various media with their children to provide them with a different perspective on sexualizing messages. Protests and other actions by groups of parents and families have been effective in confronting sources of sexualized images. Organized religious or other ethical instruction can offer girls meaningful alternatives to the values conveyed by popular culture. Girls and girls' groups can also work toward change.

Alternative media—such as feminist "zines" (web-based magazines), blogs, and other websites, as well as print-based media—can encourage girls to begin speaking out and developing their own alternatives.

"Girl power" groups can also support girls in various ways and provide important alternative influences (APA Task Force, 2007).

Consistent and empathic messages to boys are equally important, because reports of bullying and general aggression in boys are increasing. In addition, violence in boys may be viewed by many adults as normative and dismissed with such clichés as "Boys will be boys" or "He's working off steam." Although we have focused more on girls than on boys in this chapter, boys are also susceptible to media messages about male power, strength, and dominance, and to the cultural romanticizing of "bad boys." Many males are themselves vulnerable to bullying if they don't adhere to the stereotypical behaviors of young males or are viewed as "weak" or "soft" by others. When boys are portrayed in the media as only wanting involvement with girls who fit the stereotypes of contemporary beauty, they are also being manipulated into compliance and may end up feeling afraid to assert their own choices and/or feeling forced to behave in ways that may elicit feelings of guilt and shame. Peer pressure continues to be a powerful force in the life of children, and it sometimes plays havoc with what children are taught in their homes. Children these days have a lot of competing pressures to negotiate; they require support from parents/caregivers and from the schools—and more support from society at large than they are presently receiving—to develop strong and anchored views of themselves and others.

SUMMARY

In summary, the problem is not that children are learning about sex. The problem is that the sexualization of childhood is harming young children at a time when the foundations for later sexual behavior and relationships are being laid. Children are forced to deal with sexual issues when they are too young—specifically, when the way they think leaves them vulnerable to soaking up the sexual messages that surround them, and when they have few resources to resist these. Children learn to judge themselves and others on the basis of their looks and other gender-stereotypical qualities, ignoring other important ways to assess their value. The resulting objectification can undermine children's ability to have connected, caring relationships in the present, as well as caring relationships of which sex is a part in the future (Levin & Kilbourne, 2008).

Parents, other caregivers, and educators must be prepared to provide consistent, empathic guidance to children about their sexual development and must stretch their comfort zones when it comes to providing direct messages about sexuality. If caring adults don't take their rightful places in this effort, the messages children will internalize in this regard are those they receive from the media conglomerate.

There is much about childhood play that allows children to test out, pretend, and express their interests and normative curiosity. In addition, normative sexual play between children exists in exploratory, random, and playful ways. But parents must remain alert to ways in which they both model and respond to whatever sexualized play and behaviors they witness or discover.

Last, children's normative sexual play is just that: a forum for exploration. Most of the time, this play is not aggressive or harmful to either child. However, when elements of coercion, bullying, and aggression become patterns included in playful interactions between children, these behaviors must be addressed directly. One of the ways immediately available is parental guidance on the availability of TV and other sources of outside messages. Parents and other caregivers are encouraged to limit the amount of electronic play in which children engage and to maximize children's access to safe and supervised outdoor play, where creative imagination can lead to hours of pleasurable interactions between children.

CHAPTER FOUR

Assessment of Young Children with Sexual Behavior Problems

Clinical assessments of children (especially very young children) are challenging, and they have been discussed in numerous scholarly and clinical articles and books. Clearly, assessing young children needs to include a focus on developmental functioning, as well as on obtaining family, school, and other collateral information. What is certain is that the younger a child is, the less language the child has available, and the less cognitively sophisticated he or she is. Clinical efforts with very young children therefore have to include observational skills, creative engagement strategies, and alternative ways of learning about underlying issues.

When children present with sexual behavior problems, several unique factors must be considered:

1. The sexual behavior problems do not occur in a vacuum, so environmental factors must be explored and evaluated for their potential influence.
2. Family dynamics may play a part in the development of an array of problem behaviors, including focused sexually aggressive behaviors.
3. Children may have been sexually molested themselves, and their sexual behavior problems may be attempts to call attention to their plight and receive help.

4. Sexual behavior problems require structured interventions by parents or other primary caregivers, and it is important to assess whether consistent and empathic supervision will be possible in a child's immediate environment.

There are many different ways to conduct clinical assessments, including direct verbal interviews with primary caregivers and children (usually brief ones, in the case of the children). In addition, some assessments include a range of psychological testing, although no specific tests are currently available to yield information about sexual behavior problems in very young children (as opposed to older children and teens, who may be better able to report their thoughts and feelings on psychological instruments, and for whom clinicians may be better able to determine risk factors for the problem behaviors to persist). Unique challenges can occur with young children who are not verbally oriented, as well as with children who may be reluctant to admit to behavior they believe will get them into trouble. Specialized assessments may prove useful.

OUR SPECIALIZED ASSESSMENT PROCESS

Gil (2010a) and colleagues have utilized a specific assessment process called the Extended Play-Based Developmental Assessment (EPBDA) for several decades. They rely on this process to develop comfortable and trusting relationships with children, and to invite their participation in a meaningful way. In lieu of using a question-and-answer format, the EPBDA utilizes child-centered play therapy ("nondirective" strategies) as well as several play-based activities ("directive" strategies) to elicit important information about how children perceive themselves, their important relationships, and their environments. Clinicians using the EPBDA invite children to interact with them to "show or tell" what might be on their minds and utilize expressive therapies as additional tools to assess children's functioning. Thus children's spontaneous creations of artwork, stories, or specific play scenarios are given equal weight with other reliable sources of information.

Our assessment process for problematic sexual behaviors has been adapted from the EPBDA and targets children's sexual development and sexual behaviors, familial factors, and trauma history. This adapted assessment model is called the Assessment of Sexual Behavior Problems in Children (ASBPC). It is offered here as an example of an assessment model for young children who may not be able or willing to provide verbal information because of perceptual, cognitive, or linguistic limitations. In addition, by the time children are brought for mental health services, they may feel shame or guilt about their behaviors, and/or they may already have been interviewed several times by parents or other caretakers; they may thus feel hesitant about or unreceptive to verbal discussions of their sexual behavior problems.

As we have discussed in Chapters One and Two, children with sexual behavior problems can have myriad underlying factors and coexisting concerns. These may include physical or sexual abuse; witnessing domestic violence or other trauma; grief/loss; attachment issues; organic factors and developmental delays; general dysregulation and impulse control issues; and sometimes more specific coexisting issues, such as learning and attention difficulties. In addition, sexual behavior problems must be assessed contextually, because children often live in complex family systems with multiple stressors that can contribute to the development or maintenance of problem behaviors.

In some cases, children with sexual behavior problems may have trauma histories that have not been identified or addressed therapeutically; thus the assessment process can become an invaluable tool for crafting treatment paths for children and their family members. When children with such histories have been referred for treatment because of their victimization of other children, it is difficult for them to invest in changing their behaviors when their abuse has not been identified or resolved. Once their traumatic experiences can be addressed as seriously and as carefully as their hurtful actions toward others, they may be better able to sort out how their past experiences might be reflected in their current problems. In addition, after a certain amount of emotional healing, children may be more ready to engage in therapy on a cognitive level, and they may become more open to considering the feelings of other children since their own hurts have been affirmed.

Assessors of children with sexual behavior problems may conclude that it is in their best interest to receive supportive or trauma-focused therapy first, in combination with other specialized services.

FEATURES OF THE ASBPC

The ASBPC typically consists of four to eight individual sessions with a young child (more sessions may be needed for a child who requires more time or support before engaging in directive tasks). Sessions are conducted in an individual, once-weekly, 50-minute format and occur in a play therapy environment. This extended time frame (as opposed to much shorter evaluation or assessment time frames, in which clinicians meet with children once or twice to ask questions) is designed to allow the child ample time to become comfortable with the setting, the reason for being there, and the clinician.

Clinicians using the ASBPC do not initially ask children direct questions about their sexual behavior problems, but instead utilize nondirective expressive therapies to allow children to begin communicating in nonverbal ways. This process allows clinicians to gain an understanding of the children's overall functioning, with particular attention to ways in which their sexual thoughts, feelings, and behaviors compare to those of same-age peers, as well as to how these sexual thoughts, feelings, and behaviors may intrude into children's general functioning.

Clinical Intakes

The intake meeting that starts the assessment process has two primary objectives: (1) to obtain specific information from parents/other caregivers; and (2) to provide specific information, guidance, and limit-setting strategies to these adults. The clinician also engages in the following with the primary caregiver(s):

1. Identifying types of possible stimulation for the child, plus ways in which the level of stimulation in the home can be decreased (television, computers, bathrooms, bedrooms, etc.).
2. Describing ways in which the school or day care center will be involved, depending on the level of risk the child poses to other children.
3. Reviewing specific risk factors for the child and any known or suspected history of abuse, domestic violence, neglect, or other trauma.
4. Obtaining a signed parent agreement. In addition, written safety guidelines are reviewed, signed, and placed in the child's file.

In specifically assessing the sexual behavior problem(s), the clinician asks for behavioral descriptions of each problem; length of time the problem has existed; interventions that parents/caregivers have used to respond to the problem to date; their understanding of settings where the behavior occurs; and their perceptions of the child's emotional state both before and after the behavior. As mentioned previously, known or suspected histories of abuse are also discussed, as well as the child's overall social and developmental history.

One or more of the following instruments are also administered, to inform treatment focus and sequencing of interventions:

- Child Behavior Checklist (CBCL), ages 6–18 (Achenbach & Rescorla, 2001) or ages 1½–5 (Achenbach & Rescorla, 2000)
- Child Sexual Behavior Inventory (CSBI), ages 2–12 (Friedrich, 1997)
- Trauma Symptom Checklist for Children (TSCC), ages 8–16 (Briere, 1996)
- Trauma Symptom Checklist for Young Children (TSCYC), ages 5–7 (Briere, 2005)

Sequence of Assessment Activities

The following sequence of assessment activities (see Form 4.1 at the end of the chapter) is offered with the understanding that *the order and emphasis of each session should be guided by clinical judgment and the child's overall readiness for each task*, which is evaluated at the outset of the sessions.

1. Setting the context, explaining the process and session structure, and introductory nondirective tasks
2. Introduction of directive tasks:
   a. Artwork
      - Free drawings
      - Kinetic Family Drawing (K-F-D)
      - Self-portraits
   b. Sand therapy
   c. Play genograms
3. Reconstructive tasks that directly address the sexual behavior problem
4. Color Your Feelings
5. Safety review, discharge planning, and conveying preliminary recommendations

Nondirective Tasks

Play therapy has been found to be a pivotal diagnostic and treatment approach to working with children, and its applications and potential benefits have been well articulated (Gitlin-Weiner, Sandgrund, & Schaefer, 2000; Landreth, Sweeney, Homeyer, Ray, & Glover, 2005; Schaefer, 1993, 2003). Nondirective, child-centered play therapy allows the child to take the lead and guide what happens in therapy sessions. As best explained by Landreth (2012), child-centered play therapists have an unwavering commitment to providing children with unconditional acceptance and trusting that inner capacities are at their disposal to initiate their healing process. Thus our initial approach to all children is to give them an opportunity to find those reparative capacities and to show us through their play what might be on their mind. Those unfamiliar with child-centered play therapy would benefit greatly from attending workshops or reading clinical materials that provide precise guidance (Giordano, Landreth, & Jones, 2005).

Some of the nondirective introductory tasks we use in the ASBPC are child-centered play therapy, nondirective sand therapy, and free drawings. Children are allowed to interact with a play therapy environment freely, and clinicians value and learn from what they do and what they don't do. Clearly, clinicians will be able to assess these spontaneous play activities more readily with training and experience in this area.

Directive Tasks

Childhood sexual behavior problems are compelling problems that often put other children at risk. As such, these behaviors urgently require direct interventions to set firm limits and teach children alternative behaviors. Sexual behavior problems are simply not amenable to child-centered therapies alone, and although child-centered approaches provide a valuable adjunctive benefit in these cases, these problems require more specific interventions. Thus many of the directive tasks listed above (requests to participate in specific art activities, as well as to engage in play or conversation about the problem behaviors) must be incorporated with nondirective play therapy approaches to improve our understanding of children and their problems. We discuss these directive tasks in greater detail in a later section.

Assessing sexual behavior problems specifically is the most obvious departure from a child-centered approach, which gives unconditional approval. In these cases, clinicians and caretakers alike need to help children reduce their hurtful behaviors toward others.

Gathering Data and Making Recommendations

After assessments are completed, clinicians may submit full reports to the referring agencies with written recommendations, including but not limited to the following: individual, group, and/or family therapy, and/or referrals to a higher level of care if appropriate. Clinicians also meet with parents or other primary caregivers, to clarify and reinforce their future responsibilities. The caregivers may be asked to provide increased supervision and set specific limits with their children. Clinicians also guide them in developing realistic ways to increase their supervision and monitoring of their children's behaviors across settings, so that high-risk situations can be avoided or ameliorated.

Although several sessions include a schedule for presenting directive play-based activities, the context for the assessment is initially and largely nondirective. Thus a child can choose whether to engage in play prior to the task of the day, or after. If the child chooses to complete the task first, but then rushes through the directive task to get to the nondirective playtime, the sessions can incorporate a different structure (e.g., "Today you will have time to play or create for the last 15 minutes of our time together"). Clinical observations of the child's approach to play, process within the play, thematic content, and responsiveness to the clinician are as relevant to the data as directive tasks are. As mentioned previously, the more training and experience clinicians have in play therapy, the greater use of this work they can make. Ample resources are available to clinicians unfamiliar with play therapy, many of which are listed in the Resources section at the end of this book.

Termination of Assessment

When clinicians are working with children in an extended assessment that requires their attendance over weeks of individual or conjoint sessions, it becomes important and relevant to provide the children with a context for understanding how long they will spend time meeting with the clinicians and what will happen after the assessment is complete.

It is important to remind children of the final date, and to discuss time each week. The sessions can be specified in a calendar, or children can be reminded at the beginning of each session that "we have three more to go." When the conclusion of the assessment is approaching, clinicians can remind children—for example, by saying,

> "As you know, we are going to have our last meeting on [specific date], and I would like us to do a few things before then. First, I would like us to look back at when you first came here, the things we have done together, the activities you have enjoyed, and what you've learned about yourself. I would then like to give you and your [parent/caregiver] some ideas about where we go from here and what I think might be helpful for you. I would also like to plan a goodbye session and celebration, so I would like to hear how you would like to celebrate our last meeting together."

Depending on the children's age, their willingness to engage in dialogue, and their general cooperation, verbal reviews may be minimal. Instead, clinicians might present children with a little booklet with pictures and activities that were completed during the assessment, and then reveal what lies ahead.

In addition, clinicians can make some concluding comments such as these:

> "I'm grateful for your willingness to come to assessment sessions."
> "We have gotten to know each other better, and I appreciate that."
> "I appreciate your being open with your thoughts and feelings."
> "I have some ideas about how to be of help to you and your parents/
>   caregivers, and about some special issues that might need added
>   attention."

Children may or may not have difficulty with the termination session. Saying goodbye may evoke other endings or losses in their lives, some of which may not have been properly explained or processed. Children may want to express sadness or anger about ending the assessment process and may find it difficult to express these feelings directly. It may be useful to find a way for children to chronicle their feelings, such as providing a piece of easel paper on which they can write whatever they want, or asking them to choose a miniature that best shows their thoughts and feelings about ending. This session may also last a little longer than others, and it's important to emphasize that termination is a celebration of completion. When it has become clear that some children will be continuing to receive other services, it's relevant for them to be informed of that, and for parents/caregivers to be informed that a small break between this assessment process and new services might be indicated

When clinicians have a termination session with children, the goals are not only to provide closure for children as just described, but to provide feedback to children and parents (and referring professionals when necessary), to provide referrals as needed, and to provide written reports to referring professionals as required. It is particularly important for clinicians to tell children what clinical information will be shared and not shared with parents, and how they will preserve the children's confidentiality when working with their parents. Children may be encouraged to tell their parents certain important information directly, and clinicians can guide and support this process when it is useful and appropriate. When clinical recommendations include ongoing therapy with the clinician who conducted the assessment, children should be informed about how the process may or may not change. For example, if the assessment has identified anger management as an area for attention, children can be told that some of the time they will be able to lead the therapy, and at other times the clinician will address the issue of anger management. When reports of child abuse or neglect must be made, parents/caregivers may be told ahead of time about the reports, encouraged to make the reports themselves, or invited to be present while the clinician makes calls to appropriate authorities.

DIRECTIVE TASKS UTILIZED IN THE ASBPC

Artwork

Three drawing/art tasks are included in the ASBPC: (1) free drawings, (2) K-F-D, and (3) self-portraits.

Free Drawings

Free drawings can be produced by children throughout the assessment. If they like to paint or draw, they might complete them, without invitation, in the first session. During this first session, goals of child-centered play therapy are emphasized. Those goals are to establish a warm, caring, accepting relationship with a child; to give unqualified acceptance;

to create an atmosphere of safety and permissiveness (and set limits as needed); to be sensitive, empathic, and responsive to the child's feelings; to reflect feelings back to the child so that he or she can develop insight; to respect the child's capacity to act responsibly; to allow the child to lead in play and conversation; and to allow the children to set the pace.

It is important for clinicians who are not art therapists to understand that the process of making art has inherent curative properties (Rubin, 2005; Malchiodi, 1998). Thus clinicians should not talk, ask questions, or otherwise interrupt children while they draw or paint. If children talk during art making, clinicians listen but don't actively engage in conversation. It is also important to stay informed of the research on children's drawings, in order to compare and contrast important variables (Peterson & Hardin, 1997).

DIRECTIVES FOR FREE DRAWING

Clinicians can begin by saying simply, "You can draw or paint whatever you like," or "You can create anything that comes to mind." They can pose one of the following therapeutic questions *after* a child is finished with a free art activity: "Tell me about your picture," or "You can say as much or as little as you'd like about your picture."

Kinetic Family Drawing

In the K-F-D activity (Kaufman & Burns, 1972), a child is asked to draw a picture of his or her family. This drawing is thought to facilitate the emergence of the child's perceptions of relationships among family members, as well as the child's adaptive and defensive styles in relation to family functioning. The goal of the K-F-D as an assessment task is to identify the child's perceptions of self, family, and/or support system, as well as family dynamics. It is useful to keep the drawing in the child's file. If the child asks to take the drawing home after the session, it is useful to take a picture of the artwork to be maintained in the child's file, and to obtain a signed consent from the parent to take photographs of expressive art tasks.

DIRECTIVES FOR THE K-F-D

Again, the opening directive is simple: "Draw a picture of yourself and your family doing something together . . . some kind of action." A clinician may ask one or more of the following questions after the child has finished the activity:

"Tell me about your picture or drawing."

"What is going on in this picture?"

"How do the figures in the drawing feel about one another? If they could speak, what would they say to each other?"

"If the girl [boy] could speak, what would she [he] say to . . . ?"

"I wonder what this person is thinking or feeling?"

"If your family wasn't doing this activity, what else would they do?"

SPECIAL CONSIDERATIONS AND PROCESSING SUGGESTIONS

A clinician should stay at the periphery of this activity, without initiating idle chatter that distracts from or diffuses the child's engagement with the activity. The clinician should provide silent involvement and allow the drawing to proceed without interruption. Once the drawing is completed, an open dialogue in which the child volunteers a broad range of information should take place. The clinician should ask open-ended questions, being cautious not to impose value-laden words. Instead, he or she might say, "I noticed that your picture of yourself is smaller than everyone else in your drawing. Tell me more about that," or "I notice your dad is standing close to you and holding your hand," as opposed to "It seems like you and your dad are really close."

The clinician should avoid sharing interpretations, but chronicle them. Here is an example of what can go wrong with sharing interpretations:

CLINICIAN: Wow, it seems you and your dad must really like each other. He's really close, and you're holding hands.

CHILD: (*No comment.*)

CLINICIAN: What's your favorite thing about your dad?

CHILD: Nothing.

CLINICIAN: What are you and your dad doing in this picture?

CHILD: He's trying to take me to my room.

CLINICIAN: Oh, he's trying to take you to your room.

CHILD: Yeah, he hides me in there to do bad things.

The child's drawing of his father next to him and holding his hand was the child's externalization of the danger involved when the father was close enough to isolate him. The clinician's interpretation, predictably, was wrong, and this could have caused the child to abruptly shut down. Luckily, the child was able to override the therapist's interpretation to provide his own—but doing this requires a lot of ego strength (more than many children have). Thus interpretations are best avoided. Instead, describing what the clinician sees can be more useful. For example, "I notice your dad is drawn next to you and is holding your hand. What's that like for you?"

Self-Portraits

Children are offered pencils, markers, and/or paints. Young children will probably be better able to make drawings on standard-size paper with a #2 black pencil. Markers can be brought out to "color in" the picture if children wish. When easels, paints, and brushes are visible, children may ask to work with these tools; however, they may struggle more with wet paints, which can prevent them from providing more precise details and can thus cause them to feel frustrated.

The goals of self-portraits are to identify children's self-perceptions, emotions/thoughts, developmental issues, self-image/self-esteem, and areas of concern. Children with sexual behavior problems may exaggerate the genitals. If children look for more direction, clinicians should tell them that whatever they do is fine and that there is no right or wrong way of doing this drawing.

DIRECTIVES FOR SELF-PORTRAITS

Once again, the opening directive is simple: "Draw a picture of yourself." A clinician may ask one or more of the following questions after the child has finished the self-portrait:

"Tell me about your picture."
"What is going on in your picture?"
"What is this little girl [boy] thinking in this picture?"
"How does the little girl [boy] feel in the picture?"

Clinicians are encouraged to consult with a registered art therapist to develop a better understanding of self-portraits. Clinicians should maintain their role as silent observers.

SPECIAL CONSIDERATIONS AND PROCESSING SUGGESTIONS

If children refuse to make self-portraits, clinicians should move to another activity (e.g., a free drawing). It is important to avoid power struggles and emphasize to children that they can make whatever kind of picture they want, including an abstract self-portrait (older children like this). The directive for an abstract self-portrait is "Use lines, shapes, colors, or images to make a picture of you." Again, it is important to stay actively involved yet quiet, to avoid interrupting the art process or distracting children. Clinicians are advised to observe changes in children's affect as they make art, and they may comment after the fact on what they noticed. For example, a clinician could share: "I noticed that you wrinkled your forehead and moved around in your chair when you were drawing this part of the picture."

Clinical comments on any of these three types of artwork should always be directed at a picture and not a child. It is important to remain aware that one of the most valuable aspects of art is that it provides children with a "safe enough distance" from their feelings. For example, they can attribute sadness or anger to the picture they have made, without "owning" the sadness or anger for themselves. This distance may give children an opportunity to begin to process their feelings in a safe way.

Sand Therapy

The use of sand therapy is becoming more and more popular across the United States, and this popularity has emerged in tandem with ample clinical resources for its therapeutic use (Homeyer & Sweeney, 2004, 2011; Turner, 2005; Mitchell & Friedman, 1994; Carey, 1999). A professional organization (Sandplay Therapists of America) exists with the sole purpose of providing education and inspiration about a Jungian form of sand therapy, called "sandplay." More and more child therapists have become better informed and specially trained in the use of sand therapy, and recognize it as a valuable practice for helping children explore their worlds.

In the context of the ASBPC, sand therapy makes several experiences possible for children: externalization of their internal worlds; emotional and mental assimilation of difficult experiences; and projection, working through, and development of insight. The sand therapy process is evocative to self and others, and children's creations in the sand tray often allow for the integration of emotionally charged situations through the process of making something whole in a limited space.

Sand therapy is available to children at any time during the assessment process, but if they have not used it spontaneously, clinicians can ask them to participate and may even give them a directive for a specific activity in the sand.

Directives for Sand Therapy

The following directives are offered with the understanding that clinicians will use this tool to the limit of their training (and not beyond).

The opening invitation is quite simple: "Using as few or as many miniatures as you would like, build a world in the sand. There is no right or wrong way to do this, and whatever you do will be fine." Some clinicians prefer to say, "Using these miniatures, make anything you would like in the sand." Clinicians are advised to try out both directives and see which works better.

In addition to these approaches, clinicians may ask children to show them, using miniatures in the sand tray, "what your touching problem feels like to you," or "how big a problem it is in school," or "when it is likely to be a bigger or smaller problem."

After children create their sand scenarios, clinicians model observation and value what has been created. Clinicians will decide how much to talk after a sand scenario is completed, and may ask a wide range of questions or may make comments designed to cause children to be introspective about their creations.

It is usually helpful to allow for spontaneous communication from children and/or to tell them they can say "as much or as little" as they want. Useful questions/comments are open-ended invitations, such as "Tell me about your world," "Tell me what kind of world you've built," or "What is going on in your world?"

Special Considerations and Processing Suggestions

A clinician should plan and leave ample time for viewing each sand scenario. The length of time it takes to create a scenario may vary. If time is almost up, the clinician should thank the child and process the scenario at a later session with a photograph or reconstruction.

The rules of sand therapy are few. The sand stays in the tray (it is best to provide this rule once it is apparent a child needs it, rather than at the beginning of the session). In addition, the clinician does not break the plane of the tray by putting his or her hands in the tray to point at things. Finally, the clinician does not dismantle a scenario in front of a child.

Play Genograms

A "genogram" is a recognized assessment tool that allows clinicians to visualize children's family structures, to obtain demographic information, and to elicit children's perceptions of important people in their lives (McGoldrick, Gerson, & Petry, 2008). In order to use a genogram in assessing a child, a clinician is advised to draw the child's genogram ahead of time or to draw it with the child's help in session. Once the basic genogram is drawn on a large piece of easel paper, the child can be asked to include other important people or pets.

Gil (2003a, 2003b) has adapted McGoldrick and colleagues' procedure for using a genogram by adding a playful component involving the use of miniatures. After a child's genogram is drawn, the child is then asked to find miniatures that best show his or her thoughts and feelings about each family member or other significant person, including the child him- or herself. A later task is to find a miniature to represent the relationship between the child and each other person in the genogram.

A play genogram can be done individually (individual play genogram) or with members of the child's family (family play genogram). The goals of the play genogram for assessment purposes are to collect information about children's perceptions of their families and their social support systems; to expand children's ability to communicate by using symbolic language; and to allow children to express thoughts/feelings about themselves and important others.

Directives for Play Genograms

Once a child's basic genogram has been constructed, a clinician can say something like this: "What I'd like you to do now is to pick one or more miniatures that show your thoughts and feelings about everyone in the family, including yourself. Then you can put the miniature(s) in the circle or square in which it belongs."

The following are examples of some therapeutic questions to pose after the child is finished with the genogram activity:

"Say as much or as little as you want about the play genogram."
"Tell me about this [miniature]."
"What is it like for the [miniature] to _____?"
"How do [miniature A] and [miniature B] get along?"
"What would [miniature A] say to [miniature B] if it could?"
"What is the [miniature] thinking/doing/feeling?"
"How was it for you to do this activity?"

Special Considerations and Processing Suggestions

Clinicians who use play genograms are advised to allow children to choose their miniatures on their own. It is important to leave ample time for viewing and ask children to say "as much or as little" as they would like about the things they chose. Maintaining an open stance is better than using more pointed questions, such as "Can you explain the meaning of this miniature to me?" In processing a child's play genograms, it is best to try to stay within the child's metaphors as long as possible without shifting too quickly to real life. If a child has picked a wolf for his or her father, a clinician might want to say, "Tell me about the wolf," "How does the wolf spend his time?", or "Who does the wolf like to spend his time with?", rather than "How is your dad like a wolf?" However, once children begin to use first-person accounts to describe themselves or people in their genogram, clinicians can follow their lead.

Reconstructive Tasks

The goals for any reconstructive task are as follows: to help children create organized narratives of their problem behaviors, including their cognitions and emotional experiences; to assess children's understanding of the factors leading up to problem behaviors, as well as of the behaviors' impact on themselves and others; to help them begin working through the behaviors by externalizing and containing thoughts and feelings within a story that has a beginning, a middle, and an end; and to provide psychoeducation and begin orienting children to the need to correct the sexual behavior problems.

An effective reconstructive exercise gives children an opportunity to tell their stories in a way that feels relatively comfortable and unthreatening, and yet to explore the meanings they have assigned to what occurred. One of the important tasks of therapy will be to help children understand what their thoughts are and how many of these thoughts may be limiting, self-blaming, or shifting blame away from themselves to others. In CBT, such thoughts are called "cognitive distortions," and it is important to do some cognitive restructuring even at the assessment stage by giving children new information and allowing them to consider alternative explanations and understandings (Cohen & Mannarino, 1993). Moreover, when children are allowed to use art, fill in words or sentences, and/or create a scenario with miniatures, they may be less hesitant to show what happened than they often are to tell what happened.

Sometimes children can be given extra privacy—for example, by allowing them to fill in words in private, to wear a mask or sunglasses, or to get behind a puppet structure to show what happened while keeping themselves camouflaged. Such modifications sometimes lend courage to the tellers. It is important to note that for purposes of the assessment, the reconstructive tasks are designed to assess how comfortable children are with accountability, not to do therapeutic work at this time.

Directives for Reconstructive Tasks

The directives vary for each type of reconstructive activity, but the underlying expectation is that children will be able to "play out" and narrate their behaviors. Here is a sample directive to begin an activity: "This is you, this is [alleged victim] . . . show me what happens when you have the touching problem." Or, simply, "Show me what happened when [a specific incident occurred]." Again, the story can told by the child from behind a puppet screen or in some other way that the child experiences as private and safe.

For the reconstructive task we use a "cartoon narrative," and the opening directive can be as follows:

> "As you can see, I have drawn some boxes on pieces of paper that are laid out like a comic book or a cartoon. What we're going to do is to draw out what happens when you have the touching problem [or touching idea, or touching feeling]. You can tell me and I can draw it, or you can draw it if you want. You can also add words to tell what happens. First, let's pick a specific time when the touching problem occurred to draw or write about, and then let's think back to what was happening right before. In this last box, let's show what happened right after the touching caused a problem."

Clinicians can use templates or assist children in making simple line drawings in a beginning-to-end sequence. Once the simple line drawings are made, clinicians draw bubbles on each square or with each person, and then ask children to write in what people think, feel, or want to say or do.

This cartoon narrative can also be done as a reconstructive task in a dollhouse or sand tray. For children referred for a specific sexual behavior problem, the referring incident can be used as the problem presented in the scenario. However, some children will not be able to show or discuss their sexual behavior problems during the assessment process. In these cases, clinicians can assist children by writing or drawing what the clinicians know about the incidents or what parents have described. Even when children deny that the events occurred, clinicians can offer that "lots of kids have trouble admitting what happened at first."

Special Considerations and Processing Suggestions

Children may not be enthusiastic about this project, and it's helpful to present the tasks in a matter-of-fact way. Clinicians can encourage children to write in (or whisper to them what to write in) the bubbles, and to try to have the bubbles include feelings, thoughts, physical sensations, and behaviors. To get reluctant children started, clinicians can ask, "What are you feeling now?", "What are you thinking now?", or "What are you feeling in your body now?" Many children will need assistance in setting up the scenario, and drawing simple stick figures may facilitate this process. A clinician may need to take the lead by drawing a stick figure for the child client and a stick figure of the child who reported the problem behavior. The clinician can then say, "This is you . . . and this is your sister. You're in her bedroom. Mom and Dad are downstairs. You had a touching idea, and now show me what happened after you closed the bedroom door . . . "

Once the child shows the narrative, the clinician reviews the narrative, repeating what the child has said about thoughts, feelings, body sensations, and so on. For example, if a child has written, "I'm going to make him pay!" and describes feeling "angry and hurt," the clinician will narrate: "So here you are feeling hurt and angry, and you are saying to yourself, 'I'm going to make him pay.' " Again, the goals are clinical assimilation and an understanding of how thoughts can lead to feelings and feelings can lead to thoughts. Clinicians eventually try to interrupt these negative thoughts and concurrent feelings.

Color Your Feelings

The Color Your Feelings task (see Form 4.2 at the end of this chapter) is designed to assess children's experiences with diverse affect and expression, particularly as these relate to different settings or relationships with different people. Specifically, the goals for this activity are to understand and document the type of feelings that children feel "most of the time"; to help children identify more clearly the feelings they are having with particular people or in response to particular events or situations; to encourage children to understand the intensity of their feelings (i.e., to realize that some feelings are more intense than others); and to illustrate for the children ways in which certain events or situations can have a dramatic impact on emotions. Children tend to respond positively to this activity, and many of us have had the experience of children coming into therapy and asking to do a Color Your Feelings about specific persons, events, or situations.

Directives for Color Your Feelings

A child is asked, "List the feelings that you have most of the time," and the clinician or child writes the list on a piece of paper. A line is then drawn from each feeling word to a small box, and the child is asked to pick a color for each feeling on the list and color in the box, thus creating an affective color code. Once the color code is complete, the clinician offers a line drawing of two gingerbread persons (see Form 4.2) and asks the child to use the color code to show the type and intensity of feeling he or she (as one of the gingerbread figures) experiences with a particular person in a particular situation. For children with sexual behavior problems, the first directive is used to assess children's affective experience "most of the time," and then to assess how that might change when they have the "touching problem" (or "touching idea or feeling").

Clinicians may ask the following questions after children have finished the activity: "Tell me about your picture," "What do you notice about your picture(s)?", or "What do you think is the same or different between the two?" Clinicians might also make comments such as these: "It seems you feel a lot of mad feelings when you have the touching idea. Tell me about the mad feelings." Or "Your sad feeling is big when you have the touching problem, and very small most of the time. Say a little bit more about how your sad feeling grows."

Special Considerations and Processing Suggestions

As with many of the other activities described in this chapter, clinicians are advised to provide silent involvement, so that children can fully engage with the artwork without interruption. Open dialogues are usually most beneficial when children finish their tasks, and clinicians are encouraged to ask open-ended questions, again being cautious not to impose value-laden words. Instead of saying, "It looks like you've used 'dark/sad' colors for the bottom of your body," clinicians can comment, "I noticed that you have blue and gray on the bottom half of your body. Tell me about that." If younger children cannot think of the names of feelings, clinicians might have to offer some feeling cards (or ideas), so that children can identify the feelings they feel themselves.

SUMMARY

Conducting a comprehensive, child-friendly assessment of children with sexual behavior problems is challenging, as many of them either cannot articulate or are hesitant to openly discuss their thoughts and feelings. Our specialized assessment process invites children to communicate their thoughts and feelings both verbally as well as through a series of play-based activities. Building relationships with families and their children is equally important. We recognize how critical a family's guidance and support will be in helping children control impulsive, inappropriate behaviors. We also acknowledge that parental or caregiver responses can either help or hinder overall progress.

Finally, this assessment approach creates the context for the work to be done in treatment. Children learn immediately that clinicians are concerned about their sexual behavior problems and that they are willing to help in a nonjudgmental, caring, and sensitive manner. Many of these children, as previously noted, can have low self-esteem and limited social skills and may be seeking limits or guidance from parents or caregivers.

FORM 4.1 Assessment of Sexual Behavior Problems in Children (ASBPC): An Overview

PARENT INVOLVEMENT

INTAKE—PARENT REPORT MEASURES	SAFETY PLANNING WITH PARENT PRIOR TO SESSION ONE
a. Child Sexual Behavior Inventory (CSBI)	a. Review and sign "Guidelines for Parents of Children with Sexual Behavior Problems"
b. Child Behavior Checklist (CBCL)	b. Review current family, community, or school safety plan
c. Trauma Symptom Checklist for Children (TSCC/TSCYC)	

FOUR TO SIX SESSIONS WITH CHILD

SESSION 1
TASK: SETTING THE CONTEXT

Drawing Task A. Free Drawing

Nondirective Playtime

SESSION 2
TASK: SAND THERAPY

Build A World In The Sand

Drawing Task B. Kinetic Family Drawing

Nondirective Playtime

SESSION 3
TASK: PLAY GENOGRAM

Drawing Task C. Self-Portrait

Nondirective Playtime

SESSION 4
TASK: RECONSTRUCTIVE TASK
(addressing referring problem specifically)

Nondirective Playtime

SESSION 5
TASK: COLOR YOUR FEELINGS
(e.g., "talking about the touching idea/problem," "when I have the touching idea/problem.")

Nondirective Playtime

SESSION 6
TASK: CLOSURE / SAYING GOODBYE
(conveying recommendations to caregiver)

Nondirective Playtime

From Eliana Gil and Jennifer A. Shaw (2013). Copyright by The Guilford Press. Permission to photocopy this form is granted to purchasers of this book for personal use only (see copyright page for details). Purchasers can download a larger version of this form from *www.guilford.com/p/gil9*.

FORM 4.2 Color Your Feelings

My list of feelings most of the time . . . and their color.

This is where my feelings are in my body when . . .

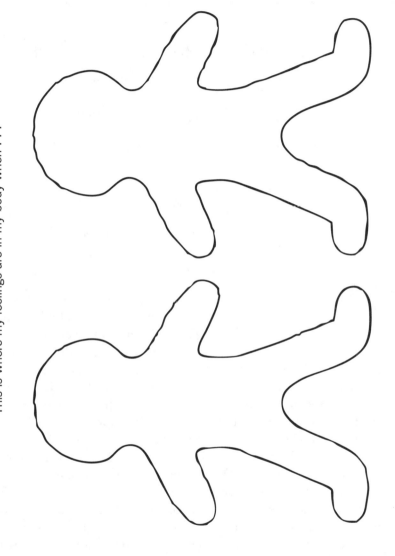

CHAPTER FIVE

Consensus-Based Treatment Areas and Suggestions for Work with Primary Caregivers

Too often, professionals have adapted the principles that guide the treatment of adult sexual offenders to working with children and adolescents who have sexual behavior problems. However, there are enormous developmental differences between children with sexual behavior problems and adult sexual offenders; the therapy provided for each age group must reflect these differences (Friedrich, 2007). Unfortunately, persisting stereotypes continue to interfere with the delivery of developmentally appropriate treatment interventions for young and school-age children: The children are viewed as victims of sexual abuse or as future sex offenders. As we have noted in Chapter One, neither stereotype is accurate for the majority of children who exhibit sexual behavior problems. Nevertheless, because of perceptions shaped by these beliefs, children often face repercussions that do not treat their underlying issues or correspond to their actions (Friedrich, 2007). Friedrich has encouraged a revised and broader set of perspectives on children's sexual behavior problems, including a focus on attachment, ego development, self-regulation, and relational issues in therapy. Attachment dynamics and family relationships have traditionally been ignored, even when they are usually the largest contributors to these problems.

CONSENSUS-BASED AREAS FOR TREATMENT

The recent research on treatment of young and school-age children with sexual behavior problems has produced the following broad consensus-based areas for treatment: (1) therapeutic attention to trauma when appropriate (with a flexible approach to integrating a focus on the trauma with a focus on the sexual behavior problems); (2) active, direct caregiver involvement in treatment; and (3) inclusion of psychoeducation and CBT-focused interventions for direct management of sexual behavior problems. In addition, several key treatment factors have been shown to promote the long-term effectiveness of therapeutic interventions. These other factors include implementing family and community controls (clear limits, safety/supervision, and limit setting) to contain the sexual behaviors and reduce the potential for further exposure to sexualized material; teaching coping skills; assisting children directly with emotional regulation; facilitating relationship building between a child and his or her primary caregiver; and building supports outside of treatment.

Consensus-Based Area 1: Therapeutic Attention to Trauma When Appropriate

A developmentally sensitive assessment prior to treatment selection (see Chapter Four) is highly recommended in order to determine the priority and sequence of treatment foci for the referred child, caregiver(s), and/or other family members. When a child presents with both a serious sexual behavior problem and a significant trauma history, important clinical questions arise. As noted by Chaffin et al. (2006), if the child is exhibiting significant trauma-related symptoms, trauma-focused treatment may be the first priority or the primary focus in interventions. For a child without significant trauma symptoms or other internalizing symptoms (e.g., anxiety, depression), an approach focused on the sexual behavior problem itself may be a better fit—especially in a case where the trauma was not proximal to the onset of the problem (Chaffin et al., 2006; Silovsky et al., 2012).

Chaffin et al. (2006, p. 18) suggest the following approach to treatment consideration and selection in cases involving trauma or other comorbid problems:

> For example, when children with SBP [sexual behavior problems] primarily suffer from serious traumatic stress symptoms, trauma-focused

[approaches are] considered, with added SBP components addressing necessary environmental changes, supervision, and self-control strategies. When SBP are one element of a broad, overall pattern of early childhood disruptive behavior problems, well-supported models such as Parent–Child Interaction Therapy (Brestan & Eyberg, 1998), The Incredible Years (Webster-Stratton, 2006), Barkley's Defiant Child protocol (Barkley & Benton, 2013), or the Triple-P program (Sanders, Conn & Markie-Dadds, 2003) might be considered, integrated with SBP specific treatment components. When the primary problem is a chaotic or neglectful family environment, interventions focused on creating a safe, healthy, stable and predictable environment may be the top priority. When insecure attachment is a major concern, short-term interventions emphasizing parental sensitivity have been found to be the most effective (Bakermans-Kranenburg, van IJzendoorn, & Juffer, 2003).

Clinical Illustration

Clinical presentations involving trauma can be varied and complex. I (J. A. S.) worked with a 10-year-old boy who started treatment 5 weeks after he was discovered in his bedroom playing a "penis game" with his 5-year-old male cousin. My client, Frankie, had asked the 5-year-old to suck his penis, and had bribed him with a video game. An assessment of my client and collateral data from an investigation on behalf of the victim determined that this was the second incident.

I first met with my client's uncle and grandparents (with whom he presently lived), and they made it clear that they expected me to find this child in need of residential treatment; they asked me for funding resources and referrals for treatment centers. The uncle admitted to being enraged. He told me that he had yelled at his nephew, grabbed him, spanked him with a belt, and then isolated him in his room until child protective services could respond to his call. Frankie had waited in his room for 7 hours, listening intently to his grandmother, grandfather, uncle, and young cousin yelling and then crying about what had occurred. He heard his uncle storm around the house for several hours, periodically recounting the incident to those who returned his call: the police, then a child protective services hotline worker, then a detective who was assigned to the case. By the time this child got to my office for an assessment (which seemed to have been arranged mainly because of the caregivers' desire for "proof" of a need for placement in a residential facility), no one had genuinely talked with him. His relatives had given him only directives to stay far away from his cousin, and he had been interviewed by a detective whose interest was primarily in exploring the "offense" and how many times he had victimized the younger boy. His punishment to date had been isolation, and he had started to withdraw.

For 5 weeks, Frankie went to school and came home to his bedroom. He was taken off sports teams, and toys were stripped from his bedroom. He watched his young cousin receive special attention, such as going on extra outings with his uncle and grandparents. His caregivers were afraid and confused; they seemed to huddle in secrecy, to talk only with one another, and to avoid and ignore Frankie.

Frankie stopped talking to peers and teachers at school. He also started wetting the bed. Although he was even more afraid and confused than his caregivers were, these feelings were mistaken for "no empathy" at the next treatment team meeting, which took place 6 weeks after the incident. As the concerns of the various adults involved swirled during this time, and they turned to each other for support, Frankie was left to his own thoughts and perceptions that the adults only cared about protecting other children from him.

When I met with Frankie's uncle, I asked questions about my client's first 5 years of development. The still-enraged uncle replied, "Does it matter? We all have bad things happen to us, but we don't do *that*!" I responded, "In order for me to help, I need to know as much as I can about the good and bad stuff that happened to Frankie, because you're right—his actions likely are an expression of something bad that happened." The uncle proceeded to tell me about all the ways, since the child was 8 years old, that he had tried to be a parent figure to Frankie (e.g., "I took him to football practices and treated him like my own son"). I felt optimistic about his obvious investment in this child and recognized (out loud) that the uncle felt betrayed by Frankie. "All this is good to know," I told him. "He's going to need a father figure, and it sounds like you've already started building a strong relationship. Sounds like the 'bad things' might have happened before he came to live with you, before he was 8."

Frankie's grandmother then stepped in and provided as many details as she could. Like the uncle, she had had no contact with her grandson for the first 7 years of his life. She had since learned that he was removed from his biological mother at the age of 2 (abuse/neglect), placed back with her 6 months later, and removed again at the age of 4 (physical abuse); after that, he had been in six foster care placements by the age of 8. He was finally placed with his grandparents, who had not known his previous whereabouts because of their estranged relationship with his mother. His grandmother recounted reports of severe neglect, physical abuse, and "suspected" sexual abuse. His mother had abused drugs and had a nearly constant flow of men in her apartment. He had also been removed from one foster care placement due to physical abuse in that home. Neither Frankie's grandmother nor Frankie himself knew who his father was. I then asked whether my client had been in therapy before and was stunned to learn that he had not.

When I met Frankie a few days later, he was quiet and made little eye contact. I asked him whether he knew why he had been brought to see me. He shook his head; he then said he had overheard that it was about what he did to his cousin, but his grandfather "just told me to get in the car because we have an appointment." The two did not speak on the way to my office. Three sessions later, I tried to administer an assessment task designed to ascertain feeling states before, during, and after the sexual behavior problem. Frankie was starting to become comfortable with me and the play therapy setting, and to look forward to our time together, but he quickly shut down when I introduced this task. He was sitting on the floor, drawing; he put his head down and did not speak for a few minutes. I put the task away and sat with him, silently. I then offered, "This is hard stuff. I know you were hurt by a lot of people when you were even smaller than your cousin. I also know that no one helped you back then. In fact, they kept hurting you." Frankie continued lying on the floor silently, but he was clearly listening. "So I'm wondering how it feels that you are coming to see me because you hurt someone, not because you were hurt. . . . Where were all these people when you were getting hurt?"

He nodded, and then immediately started crying. I knew then that I was not going to gain his investment in preventing harm to another child until his trauma history was addressed. I postponed the referral request (to address the sexual behavior problem) and began pursuing an integrative, family-focused approach—starting with establishing safety in the home, educating Frankie's caregivers, and debunking myths about what the sexual behavior would mean about him and for him as he matured. Subsequent treatment included an emphasis on his victimizing behaviors, after he had an opportunity to process the origins of the sexual behavior problem (his own abuse).

Consensus-Based Area 2: Active, Direct Caregiver Involvement in Treatment

Outcome studies consistently identify caregiver involvement in treatment (i.e., joint parent–child sessions, separate groups for parents and children, and/or parent supportive therapy) as the program component most strongly associated with reducing sexual behavior problems in young and school-age children (Chaffin et al., 2006). In fact, Silovsky et al. (2012) assert that "current practices of treating children with sexual behavior problems as the primary problem in individual therapy or in inpatient or residential care facilities without significant caregiver involvement during treatment or aftercare are brought into question by these results" (p. 406). Friedrich (2007) has emphasized the importance of primary relationships in both the origins and treatment of these problems:

> These children first learn to relate in a disturbed manner, and subsequently use this model of relationships in their interactions with other children. Altering the first model of relating can make a difference in how these children will relate to others, and I believe this is the most efficacious form of intervention. (p. 4)

The treatment research summarized in Chapter One links both the short- and long-term effectiveness of therapy for sexual behavior problems to the participation of a parent or active caregiver. As we have noted in that chapter, the caregiver involved in treatment can be a biological parent, a kinship caregiver, or a foster parent. The preference is for a caregiver who is actively involved in the child's current daily life—ideally, a current primary caregiver who will retain full caregiving responsibilities for the foreseeable future. This caregiver must be able to stabilize the child's home environment and address contributing/maintaining factors as recommended by Chaffin et al. (2006) and Silovsky et al. (2012). As with other severe behavior problems, in order to reach the goal of reducing the intensity and frequency of the problem behavior, it is also critical to create consistency across the child's environments; this will enable the caregiver to "support and reinforce adaptive behavior, teach appropriate behavior, and provide developmentally appropriate consequences to behavior problems" (Silovsky et al., 2012, p. 406).

The more robust programs examined by Chaffin et al. (2006) include an active caregiver component. Whereas some involve caregiver support or caregiver-mediated approaches (e.g., parent skill training), others have parents/caregivers serve as active participants or partners in their children's treatment (Brestan & Eyberg, 1998; Deblinger & Heflin, 1996; Hembree-Kigin & McNeil, 1995). Chaffin et al. (2006) suggest that the most effective treatments take a focused, goal-directed approach to sexual behavior problems and educate caregivers in practical behavior management and relationship-enhancing skills (e.g., as described by Patterson et al., 2002).

Across those effective treatments reviewed by Chaffin et al. (2006), the use of the following caregiver-focused components was found: clear explanations and directives for behavior modification; specific praise for desired behaviors and attention to positive behaviors; time out as a consequence for younger children; logical, natural consequences with older children; and promotion of parental warmth, consistency, and sensitivity. In addition, direct and active caregiver involvement in outpatient treatment supports caregivers in establishing safety and supervision guidelines; monitoring for adherence to those guidelines (ongoing assessment of risk to other children, including siblings); and, once again, working to create a safe and nonsexualized environment for the children being treated. Concurrent or collateral sessions for caregivers, in-home family therapy, and parent–child dyadic sessions are some specific approaches for gaining and fostering caregivers' involvement in treatment (Chaffin et al., 2006). In randomized trials, two group therapy approaches (Bonner et al., 1999; Pithers & Gray, 1993; Pithers et al., 1998) included active caregiver involvement within the children's group and/or in a separate parent support group, as noted in Chapter One.

Active caregiver investment in treatment provides opportunities to educate families about the need to revise rules about sexual behavior and revisit expectations around boundaries (see Form 5.1 at the end of this chapter). Within dyads, or in separate sessions, treatment is furthered when clinicians can directly address expectations for children's behavior and emphasize caregivers' need to actively promote respect for privacy and modesty among all family members—not only in order to create a nonsexualized environment (Chaffin et al., 2006), but also to begin to model and practice more appropriate expression of needs and emotions.

Clinical Illustration

I (J. A. S.) worked in a group with a 6-year-old girl, Molly, whose mother suspected sexual abuse by her father (prior to the age of 4½ years).

Molly had participated in trauma-focused individual therapy prior to placement in a group with similar-age peers who presented with sexual behavior problems. Molly was referred for specialized services follow-ing her mother's unsuccessful attempts to contain or redirect Molly's masturbatory behaviors at home and school. School reports included "excessive rubbing against her chair, with refusal or inability to stop when redirected." The mother reported that Molly often masturbated at home with the same intensity and inability to be redirected: "She goes into this zone, puts her hand down her pants, and it's like she can't hear me when I tell her to do that in private." Molly's mother was very anxious and concerned about these behaviors, and eager for guidance on how she could assist and support her daughter emotionally while directly addressing the behavior, which seemed to affect Molly's self-esteem and her academic and social development.

Molly and her mother entered concurrent group therapy. During the first phase of treatment—establishing safety; defining and establishing boundaries; and reviewing and resetting family rules about privacy and modesty—Molly's mother received psychoeducation about normative and atypical sexual behaviors, and was provided with concrete parent-ing strategies to help Molly at home. Armed with this information, Mol-ly's mother was able to advocate for Molly and to request other "help-ers" at school (the school counselor was chosen as the most available, empathic, and willing person). In the child group with similar-age peers, Molly's "touching problem" was named and discussed in a developmen-tally appropriate way. The way her touching problem affected others was framed as a boundary issue: Molly was told that touching of pri-vate parts was a behavior that needed to be kept private, because it cre-ated uncomfortable feelings for those around her. The problem was also framed as an issue that "gets in the way" or "gets me in trouble." The group members talked openly about how their touching problems made it difficult to make and keep friends, and caused them to feel weird, bad, or different. Sexual feelings, particularly stimulation when sexual body parts are touched, were framed simply as natural physical responses.

Developmentally appropriate examples about how different body parts respond to touch (or the idea of touch), and how those responses are natural and predictable, were provided to Molly and her peers. For example, I offered:

> "When the doctor hits your knee [I demonstrated] to check your leg reflex, and you 'kicked,' is the kicking 'bad' or 'wrong,' or just

what bodies do? That's right. Bodies do what bodies do, and no one would feel embarrassed about having that reflex. No one would say, 'I *can't* believe her knee did that. How weird.' Because the body did what it was supposed to do. It's the same with private parts. It's a reflex that has a good feeling."

When Molly's experience was normalized, she was able to start seeing herself as someone who had a "touching feeling" that sometimes overwhelmed her—a problem that she could learn to manage. We then taught Molly that her job was learning how to identify and shrink the problem feeling so that it was not acted out in her behavior. The Affective Scaling Worksheet and the Body Thermometer (Forms 5.2 and 5.3, respectively, at the end of the chapter) were used to help Molly grasp these concepts.

Molly was much more interested in hearing how her peers shared the same problematic feelings and behaviors than in my own education about body parts. Group members talked about the places and times they could explore their private parts, and Molly and her mother learned that most children explore their bodies, but that most kids after the age of 6 learn to touch private parts out of others' sights.

Next we began to examine the origins of the touching problem, so that the intensity of Molly's feelings could eventually be affirmed and understood ("Kids whose private parts are touched inappropriately often have bigger touching ideas and touching problems than those kids whose private parts are respected"). New boundary rules for the family were created (in parent–child dyadic review), and Molly's mother learned how to redirect Molly while acknowledging Molly's distress in those moments. Together, Molly and her mother (like the other children and parents in the parent–child group review) created specific plans for home and for school. Molly's mother was her "at-home helper," and the school counselor mentioned earlier was her "at-school helper."

Specific helpful interventions were also discussed and practiced at home. For example, Molly's increasingly empowered mother more confidently approached Molly when she started masturbating at the table or while watching television. Molly was helped to notice that the touching feeling had grown to the point where it made her mom feel uncomfortable, and that she needed to stop touching in public. Molly was encouraged to find a private place, and she soon began to understand that touching in front of others was inappropriate. Molly was able to accept this limit because her mother had also told her that she understood how these thoughts and behaviors were related to past abuse. Molly and her mother worked on ways to "postpone" touching (setting a 5-minute timer while doing something active together, then revisiting the feeling to see whether it had "grown" or "shrunk" following the activity or distraction). They had practiced using Forms 5.2 and 5.3 twice during each session, so the dyad could now easily and immediately convey the intensity of the feeling. That is, Molly could say, "My touching feeling is a 3 (I want to touch)," or her mother could say, "Looks like your touching feeling is growing from a 4 to a 5. Let's do something together and see if it shrinks after a few minutes." Molly was starting to see her mother as an ally, and her mother was becoming an active and knowledgeable partner rather than a helpless observer of her daughter's maladaptive coping. The mother's anxiety was visibly reduced by the end of this first phase of treatment.

It is important to note that primary caregivers and clinicians discuss the caregivers' thoughts and feelings about masturbation and decide together on the primary messages to send children. On occasion, caregivers believe that masturbation is sinful and cannot tolerate giving their children a message that it's OK to engage in it, either in public *or* in private. In these cases, we help the caregivers set the limits they wish to set, and we may take some time to discuss with our clients how they think or feel about the limits that have been set at home. When we don't have a consensus from caregivers in a group about how to approach this subject, clinical work may be done in individual sessions with children.

In the second phase of Molly and her mother's treatment, Molly and her peers completed play-based activities designed to externalize and contain the "touching problem" (via sand therapy), to help the children learn and practice impulse control (via CBT strategies), and to help them gain insight into the origin and maintenance of the problem. During the sand therapy task (externalization and containment), Molly chose a miniature mermaid (a miniature she often used in her sand trays during individual therapy) to represent her "touching problem." The mermaid was placed in the center of the sand tray (each child had her own small sand tray and set of miniatures to choose from). With her mermaid in the center of the tray, Molly stated that she had chosen it "because I have to squeeze my legs tight together so I don't touch." Molly and her peers were then given this directive: "Now choose miniatures that can help the touching problem, or things that can be used to keep the problem small." Molly chose four miniatures and placed them around her mermaid miniature. She selected a parent figure ("my mom"); a stop sign ("I can do it later"); a fence structure around the mermaid ("so it doesn't go anywhere"); and a bicycle ("I can ride my bike").

In the parent group, Molly's mother completed a similar sand therapy project in which parents were asked to choose a miniature for their child's touching problem, as well as miniatures to show how they could help keep the problem contained. Molly's mother chose a miniature of a small, sad child (sitting with her head down, withdrawn) for the problem, and five miniatures to show how she could be Molly's helper to keep the problem small: a book ("because I'm learning better ways to help"); a mother–child figure ("because I will always love her no matter what"); a key ring ("I can give her boundaries and structure"); a small toy ("lots of things we can do together when the touching feeling grows"); and a mailbox ("I want her to know she can always talk to me").

After children and their primary caregivers work in separate groups with their peers, they come together to have an opportunity to share what they have worked on. When Molly and her peers joined the adults' group, they were all eager to share their sand trays with their caregivers. Molly sat next to her mother, and the two shared "as much or as little as they wanted" about their projects. Just like most kids in this type of treatment, Molly was proud of her sand tray, but even more eager to hear what her mom had to say. Molly's mother went through each miniature and explained how she was ready and willing to support Molly lovingly, so "you don't ever have to feel sad alone. With all these things, and your ideas too, we will keep this problem small." I remember Molly giggling and her mother tearing up as the two noticed how their collective strengths, resources, and tools overpowered the "problem," which was now named, miniaturized, and placed in a container that they could both see was full of resources.

Consensus-Based Area 3: Psychoeducation and CBT-Focused Interventions for Direct Management of Sexual Behavior Problems

CBT-focused interventions and psychoeducation for children with sexual behavior problems and their caregivers constitute a third treatment area that has received support across studies of effective treatment programs for children under the age of 12 years. This area of treatment includes teaching coping skills, providing skills to regulate affect, helping children with self-control and problem-solving strategies, and providing direct interventions (such as "stop and think before acting"). According to Chaffin et al. (2006), "Although short-term outpatient CBT . . . may not be the best option for each and every child with [sexual behavior problems], the findings do suggest that short-term outpatient CBT approaches, with appropriate parent or caregiver involvement, can be expected to yield excellent and durable results in most cases" (p. 16).

As noted earlier, children with sexual behavior problems have been successfully treated with trauma-focused CBT (TF-CBT), which is a treatment for the effects of trauma (specifically, child sexual abuse) and includes specific components for sexual behavior problems (Cohen & Mannarino, 1996, 1997; Cohen, Mannarino, & Deblinger, 2006; Deblinger, Stauffer, & Steer, 2001; Stauffer & Deblinger, 1996). According to Silovsky et al. (2012), such treatment has been found to be more effective than the passage of time, dynamic play therapy, and nondirective supportive treatment.

As emphasized by the ATSA Task Force (Chaffin et al., 2006), the cognitive and social aspects of child development must be taken into consideration by clinicians who are integrating CBT into specific treatment approaches for children with sexual behavior problems. For example, younger children may be less able than older children or adolescents to comprehend and apply cognitive coping strategies; as illustrated above in the case of Molly, they may have learned to rely on behavioral strategies such as touching their own genitals for self-soothing purposes (White, Halpin, Strom, & Santilli, 1988). Therefore, it is more appropriate for developmentally or chronologically younger clients with sexual behavior problems to be actively redirected by trusted adults to use alternative coping skills that are simpler, less reliant on cognitive processes, and more concrete, as described above in Molly's case.

In addition, young children's developmental limitations may compromise the sorts of cognitive processes involved in initiating and maintaining a sexual behavior/misbehavior (Chaffin et al., 2006). These young clients are much less able than adolescents (and certainly less able than adults) to engage in planning, grooming, rationalizing, or ignoring/recognizing cognitive distortions and "thinking errors" (often key concepts for adolescent and adult offenders' treatment programs).

Thus, typical adult sex offender treatment concepts such as learning about a cycle of sexual behaviors or correcting elaborate cognitive

distortions are far less applicable, if not inappropriate, for young children. Children have shorter attention spans and more limited impulse
control. In contrast to some adult sex offenders, childhood [sexual
behavior problems] are more likely to be impulsive rather than compul-
sive. (Chaffin et al., 2006, p. 19)

In addition, young children's cognitive age is suited to learning simple or
concrete rules about sexual behavior, but they may not grasp the abstract
reasons why such rules are important. Young children learn better by
concrete, simple demonstration, with opportunities for practice and consistent reinforcement, than by discussing concepts and applying these
to hypothetical or abstract situations. Therefore, effective interventions
for younger children emphasize modeling appropriate behaviors; setting clear external limits; and practicing new, acceptable, or appropriate behaviors across the children's environments (e.g., home, school). In
addition, expressive therapies, such as art or play therapies, may enliven
and engage children in meaningful introspection and change (Drewes &
Cavett, 2012).

For children over the age of 10 who have sexual behavior problems,
abstract principles are becoming more accessible, and hence some more
sophisticated cognitive coping strategies can be introduced. Nevertheless, their understanding of abstraction is still far less than that of adolescents or adults (Chaffin et al., 2006; Silovsky et al., 2012).

As noted earlier, psychoeducation of both children and parents is a
desirable and necessary component of treatment of children with sexual
behavior problems and their families. However, the content of psychoeducation may vary from program to program. It appears, for example,
that behavioral models of parenting are often incorporated into CBT
programs (e.g., a focus on behavioral conditioning). Other parenting
models, such as Child Parent Relationship Therapy (Landreth & Bratton, 2006), may also be helpful and easy to integrate.

Inevitably, parent/caregiver psychoeducation will be guided by the
orientation of program providers, but guidance is currently available
with adequate examples of content areas (see, e.g., Blaustein & Kinniburgh, 2010).

We have created and implemented a program called the Boundary
Project (described briefly in Chapter Six). Our program incorporates the
content areas discussed in the remainder of this chapter into groups for
parents and other caregivers, and we have articulated and prioritized
treatment components.

SUGGESTIONS FOR WORKING WITH PARENTS/CAREGIVERS

Working with parents or other primary caregivers is generally among the most critical aspects of any general child-focused work; it is especially relevant and necessary in work with sexual behavior problems. The reasons for this are clear: Young children are greatly affected by their primary caregivers' affective style and language; caretaking and nurturing; and limit setting, supervision, and guidance. If any of these areas are compromised, children can become affectively agitated or constricted, attention-seeking or withdrawn, and they can act out in order to obtain the structure most associated with children's ability to develop internal controls and self-regulate. Simply put, children develop their psychological, social, and emotional health contextually, and they are dependent on adults' healthy, empathic, warm, and informed caretaking responses. When parents or other caregivers are themselves dysregulated, are unable to take care of their own needs, have ambivalent or negative feelings about parenting, or have limited views of their own parental capacities or competencies, children suffer the consequences. In many ways, children reflect their environments. Severely traumatized children who have suffered intense, acutely painful experiences can nevertheless be positively influenced by stable, healthy, attuned primary caregivers. Conversely, distanced, conflicted, uncertain, or self-involved caregivers can have a negative impact on or interfere with the treatment outcome of abused children.

Working with parents or other caregivers of children with sexual behavior problems is remarkably challenging because these adults often have myriad feelings about the behavior problems, including confusion, worry, shame, guilt, or distress. These feelings can cause them to hide, deny, or minimize their children's behavior. Many caregivers fear other people's assumptions, judgments, possible rejection, and/or other reactions elicited by sexuality in general and children's sexual behavior problems in particular.

The components of treatment for parents or parental figures of children with sexual behavior problems include engaging the parents/caregivers in treatment; securing their cooperation; providing psychoeducation; obtaining their agreement to provide supervision; offering clear directives about parental responses; strengthening the parent–child relationship; and encouraging role modeling and co-regulation. In our Boundary Project model, these treatment tasks are accomplished within the context of a structured assessment process; a parallel treatment format for parents/caregivers and their children; and provision of a comprehensive, structured, family-based program.

Engaging Parents/Caregivers in Treatment

The first and most important task in working with parents or other primary caregivers is to engage them and obtain their investment in the therapy process; they must be convinced that their child's positive outcome depends on their participation. Depending on a clinician's theoretical orientation and approach, the child may be seen alone, in conjoint parent–child or sibling sessions, or in full family therapy sessions. Often caregivers are under the impression that since the child is the one with the identified problem, the child is the only client in therapy. Although direct clinical interventions with children who have developed particular behavioral problems is most certainly indicated, treating the family system (in other words, providing contextual or relational interventions) is usually considered not merely germane but critical to the success of treatment.

As we have noted in Chapter Four, a clinician conducts a comprehensive intake to obtain developmental and psychosocial information—in particular, to learn about the type and persistence of the sexual behavior problem, when it began, how it was discovered, where it was or is observed, and what solutions have been attempted. At one point, caregivers are invited to collaborate in the formation of treatment goals and objectives. The extent of the "buy-in" they demonstrate to the therapy process, and their stated willingness to follow clinical directives, are usually respectable predictors of positive outcome.

There are several challenges to overcome during assessment and the early sessions of treatment, because parents or other primary caregivers of children with sexual behavior problems may view therapy as a chore, an obligation, or an external requirement (e.g., it may be mandated by a school as a prerequisite for a child's return). Often the referral of a child with such a problem occurs because the child's behavior is a concern to someone in the child's life—be it a foster parent, a teacher or other school staff member, a day care provider, or the parent of another child who has disclosed the problem. The referral can also come from a court or a child protection or probation agency, in which clear mandates have been established for compliance with treatment. In addition, we have seen a number of situations in which blended families encounter inappropriate sexual acting out by one youngster against another; indeed, personal boundaries may be unfamiliar, unset, unclear, and/or confusing among children in such families. In these cases, family members can feel pitted against one other and may feel as if they need to take sides. The parent of the child with an identified sexual behavior problem may want to minimize or explain away what has occurred, while the parent of the child who may have been victimized may feel outraged and frightened. One parent may thus be more supportive of therapy than the other.

Engaging parents/caregivers who are in crisis, and who on top of that are feeling compelled to receive services they don't understand or value, is the first order of business. Over the years, we have found some areas of greater success, and we pass these along with humility—not as all-inclusive, but as a basis for your consideration.

Joining has always been an important first step. I (E. G.) can honestly say that as I listen to caregivers' stories, I focus on anything they say that I can empathize with and respond to with sincere validation. I often make affirmative statements about my understanding of their current plight—for example, "I know how you feel. I hate doing something that someone else is telling me I have to do." I also make positive and true statements such as "No one likes to be told that they don't understand their children," or "Sounds like you've got some great ideas about what will help, but no one is listening." I make sure that I am respecting caregivers' expertise about their own child, and I ask them to tell me what their ideas are about what might have precipitated the concerns. My most often-repeated statement is "I need your help to help your child." I also reassure caregivers that their love and concern for their child are obvious and necessary to successful therapy outcome.

I also help parents/caregivers focus on how the sexual behavior problems are a predicament to them at this moment. They might initially focus on the fact that their child has been suspended or expelled from school (this even happens to preschoolers who exhibit sexual behavior problems, even over very minor things such as trying to kiss classmates), or that their adult friends are forbidding play dates between their children. It's important for clinicians to try to address the problems that caregivers have in the forefront of their minds first, regardless of what these are. If clinicians can establish themselves as people who can provide real help, they are much more likely to elicit receptivity to more general clinical feedback.

The most useful approach is to convey clinical willingness to be of assistance by providing purposeful feedback about how parents or other caregivers can provide guidance and limit setting within the context of a warm and predictable parent–child relationship. Caregivers of children with sexual behavior problems often need to express their underlying fears. Most typically, these adults worry that their children will grow up to be adult sex offenders and/or will grow up to be homosexual (if the sexual behavior problems are occurring with children of the same gender). They may also harbor fears that these early sexual interests in their children could signal the development of promiscuous or otherwise deviant sexual behaviors. There is a great deal of emotionally charged misinformation about childhood sexuality, which makes the provision of psychoeducation a required element of therapy. Clinicians are well advised to inform themselves about the latest research on sexual development in children, so that they will be better able to provide some general guidelines and directions not only about contemporary normative sexual development, but about ways to understand the emergence of what might be considered non-normative or sexual behavior problems. (Incidentally, it seems paradoxical that in a country such as the United States, which appears to have an intense focus on sexuality in general, factual information on childhood sexuality remains elusive.)

"Therapeutic engagement" is the process of listening, of empathizing, and of trying to understand the parents'/caregivers' point of view, no matter what it may be—a progression of connecting with the clients and developing a respectful and helpful relationship where trust can grow. After the engagement phase, treatment goals and plans are articulated, and interventions are selected to advance those goals. During treatment, clinicians make more direct efforts to change rigid thinking patterns or clarify cognitive errors in thinking—but only after ensuring that the clients will be receptive to clinical guidance, not when they are feigning compliance or trying to get themselves stabilized in an unfamiliar therapy situation. Engagement is probably the most pivotal factor in clinical work, and once it is established, challenges can be met with less difficulty.

Securing Parents'/Caregivers' Cooperation

As mentioned above, engagement initially overrides other clinical interventions, especially during assessment. However, once a clinician has gathered data suggesting that caregivers' perceptions and attitudes are negatively affecting a child or limiting necessary support to the child, the clinician needs to challenge these adults gently in the hopes of creating more flexible responses.

Clinical Illustration

I (E. G.) worked with a father who came from a country where male strength and self-reliance were highly valued. This father had little trouble with the fact that his son had aggressively forced himself on top of a girl and humped her while holding her mouth shut. I remember him saying that "boys will be boys," and that "in this country [the United States], everything is exaggerated; nothing is just normal." I listened with interest to him talking about normative sex play in his country, and I suggested to him that childhood sexuality appears to be the same in most countries: It is not talked about publicly. He agreed that this was true when I asked him how he himself had learned about sexuality. Eventually, as he became more and more relaxed about our conversation (I had purposely avoided arguing with him or taking an opposing position at this time), I asked him to come up with times that he himself had engaged in normative sex play with peers; he had many examples. I listened intently without much comment, and this man enjoyed recalling his youth freely. When he was finished, I noted that he had described a lot of activities, but that I had not heard him describe covering someone's mouth so that they wouldn't yell or telling someone that he would kill them if they told about the activity. He looked stunned and was unable to offer a response (he was, thankfully, at a loss for words).

We had a few more appointments, now clearly with mutual trust and empathy. These enabled us to have a discussion of some beliefs that led the father to reject his son when the son admitted to having been sodomized by an older boy against his will. When the father found out about this, his behavior changed toward his son. He confided in me that he had lost respect for him, that he now saw him as "weak" and "passive," and that his wife was to blame for this softness. Once his son was able to admit to his parents that he had indeed been molesting the (much younger girl) in his neighborhood, the father appeared to take pride in the fact that the boy was sexual with a girl, not a boy. "You see," he insisted, "that was more normal than letting a boy overtake him and do with him what he wished."

Clinical dialogues with this family became very difficult at times, as I tried to explain child sexual abuse to the father and as I tried to alert him to the fact that his rejecting behaviors affected his son more than he knew. I emphasized the fact that he was in a unique position to help his son; that he was someone the son completely admired; and that he alone had a significant contribution to make to his son's development and to his son's future. This seemed to work, partly because the father had felt shame about his son and needed to feel valued by the professionals now treating his family, and partly because the father's role had been challenged when he was court-ordered to attend therapy. He seemed reassured when I elevated his status as a helper, and he responded accordingly. Once he was convinced that he alone had the power to help his son heal and move on from the abuse, the father began to relax in his attitudes. He even acknowledged that his son's abuser was indeed that! The abuser had isolated his son, applied brute force, threatened him, and hurt him physically and emotionally.

Although the father never shifted his view about crying (a sign of true weakness to him), eventually he was able to listen to his son ask for forgiveness for not being able to resist his rapist. (This seemed to be a critical request from the child's point of view, akin to a kind of confession. This child articulated this question without feeling that he needed forgiveness, but more out of respect for his father and their culture.) The father put his son's head on his shoulder (as they sat together on the couch) and softly said, "It's OK, son, that boy took advantage. He picked someone who was much smaller and younger. He was afraid to pick on someone his own size. He is weak to fight like that." The father also heard that initially his son had kicked the older boy and run from him, and the father gave him praise for that also. "Good for you, kicking that boy hard. Good for you, bruising him up. You did good, son; I am proud." Only this boy's father could give him the gift of letting him know that he had not disappointed his father and that the father was not permanently ashamed of him. For his part, the father was able to find a place of forgiveness through having the opportunity to explore all his reactions freely, without being told they were unacceptable. He was also receptive to being given his "proper place" by his son as someone who could restore his son's sense of balance and as someone who had the ultimate power to forgive. Importantly, the father confided that "My culture thinks one way, and sometimes now I think the other," acknowledging that some of his beliefs had been challenged and he had developed a more flexible understanding of the values instilled in him during childhood. He also acknowledged that his son was being raised "with the good and bad of the United States"—an influence that he had not had growing up.

Working across cultures requires sensitivity to parents'/caregivers' cultural values, while challenging their origins and exploring them in a new context. Unique situations may require revisions to previously held beliefs. In exploring childhood sexuality with parental figures, it is quite important for them to articulate their cultural context, given that many perceptions and beliefs are formed early and may not be challenged until specific situations emerge in a person's own life. These conversations need to be conducted in a nonpolarizing way, and yet clinicians may need to intervene with research findings about cultural mores as well as cultural history. Clinicians are advised to explore the history of childhood at large and to integrate some of what we know about this history into a provocative therapy dialogue designed to cause introspection. Most caregivers are shocked to hear about an ancient Roman law that gave parents the right to sell, abandon, mutilate, or otherwise dispose of their offspring, or that the practice of infanticide was practiced routinely as a tool for gender selection or population control. Regardless of which culture is being discussed, these tend to be fruitful dialogues.

Providing Psychoeducation on Issues Relevant to a Healthy Parent–Child Relationship

Early clinical efforts that engage family members in a therapy relationship, elicit meaningful parental investment in therapy, and gently challenge old attitudes and beliefs may earn the clinician the right to provide psychocducation. Earning the confidence of clients is a necessary prerequisite to offering them facts, concepts, approaches, and guidance. If purposeful efforts are not made to earn this right to be heard and to have their guidance valued, psychoeducators can work very hard to give their best advice and directives—only to have caregivers tune them out, ignore their advice, and generally look the other way.

The best way to earn the right to be heard is for clinicians to afford others the same respect that they want themselves as teachers or guides. It's important to know what parents or other primary caregivers want to hear about, what they think is important, and what they might find particularly helpful in their situation. Giving them a chance to state their needs (and then address these) is necessary and fruitful. After parental needs are understood and are used to alter or redefine a psychoeducational agenda, trust is solidified and receptivity increases. In group treatment, every group sets a slightly different agenda, and yet psychoeducation for caregivers of children with sexual behavior problems usually includes a core set of topics that cannot be omitted. Over time, as these adults come to view the clinician and the treatment as resources in their lives (as opposed to an inescapable obligation or another required step to regain control), they can more readily reflect upon, accept, and integrate the information that is delivered.

Psychoeducation for parents/caregivers of children with sexual behavior problems will touch on the topic of childhood sexuality by necessity. However, it must also include contextual information about improving or enhancing parent–child relationships.

Obtaining Parents'/Caregivers' Agreement to Provide Supervision

One of the core beliefs in work with children who have sexual behavior problems is that the children's internal controls are not working sufficiently to override their inappropriate behaviors, whether these behaviors are impulsive or planned. Because of that core belief, it becomes crucial to ensure that a child's parents or other primary caregivers are willing and able to provide mechanisms of constant supervision; this supervision becomes the child's temporary external controls. It is also important to define "supervision" as within-eyesight supervision at all times. Caregivers will find this quite demanding of their time and a real departure from their regular everyday routines. And yet obtaining a firm contract about this, while children are in treatment, is a critical key to success.

A parent who had participated in our program for about 3 months had begun to relax her supervision as she took great comfort in changes in her son's behaviors, his open sharing about his sexual behavior problems (a truly remarkable change, given his initial denials), and her growing trust that the problem was being addressed and had shown itself responsive to interventions and supervision. She was stunned, therefore, when her daughter came to her while she was cooking and said that her brother had come into the bathroom while the daughter was in there urinating: "I told him to leave, Mom, I told him, and he wouldn't!" When this mother approached her son with great concern and frustration in her voice, the boy said, "Well, she's supposed to be locking the door all the time." He then added that although he stood at the door when his sister was yelling for him to get out, he never entered the bathroom and thought his sister's reactions were funny. This child appeared to be telling his mother that he still needed external controls (he needed to be watched, and his sister needed to lock the door) in the home. The mother heard the message "loud and clear," and went back to her more structured and vigilant approach to supervision until her son developed better internal controls.

Offering Clear Directives about Parental/Caregiver Responses

Probably one of the most consistent issues that we see in parents/caregivers of children with sexual behavior problems is the adults' own discomfort with the area of childhood sexuality, their reluctance to approach the topic head-on, and their confusion about what to say or do when confronted with their children's inappropriate behaviors.

This hesitancy about addressing childhood sexual problems directly is firmly anchored in a lack of education and preparation for parents/caregivers in this general area of life. Parental figures typically struggle to find the motivation to talk with their children about normative sexual development, and even when they feel obligated and compelled to talk with them, they don't know what words to use or what messages to send. These difficulties can increase when adults are suddenly confronted with behaviors that cause them to feel concerned or ashamed. Children and teens continue to get most of their information about sexuality from conducting their own "research" (e.g., on the Internet), from self-discovery, from peers, or from other avenues of information. Rarely do adults provide enough information regarding normative sexual development, and the emphasis in what information they do provide seems to be on what *not* to do versus what is appropriate and expectable.

Because of this situation, one of our earliest interventions is to provide language that parents/caregivers can use to make the sexual behavior problems explicit, followed by ideas for setting limits and consequences. Clearly, it is important for them to provide alternative behaviors as well. Clinical role playing is often quite helpful, so that caregivers can make attempts to communicate clearly and remain aware that their nonverbal communication also needs monitoring. They need to recognize that their words are not the only information they are conveying; they also communicate with their tone of voice, intonations, facial expressions, and physical posture. Getting caregivers to be firm and gentle at the same time can feel quite challenging to them. Clinical demonstration as well as practice can help this seem more natural and increase their confidence in how to respond.

Given that the topic of childhood sexuality in general, and sexual behavior problems specifically, can arouse strong negative or conflictual thoughts and feelings, among the earliest topics to be openly addressed are normative sexual development and what is known about baseline behaviors of children across the developmental span. Most of the time, caregivers are surprised and relieved to learn that "normal" children also have overt sexual curiosity and behaviors.

Strengthening the Parent–Child Relationship

The parent–child relationships that we have seen in our clinical practice over the years have included widely varying degrees of attachment, emotional connection, positive regard and respect, and mutual nurturing. In other words, some of the relationships we encounter are "temporarily under construction" and have obvious areas that require repair. Sometimes vulnerabilities that existed before the emergence of sexual behavior problems are exacerbated by the stress or crises elicited by children who develop or maintain sexual behavior problems. At other times, preexisting relationships may have been strong, but they come under siege from the sudden and distressing loss of trust, respect, and positive regard between family members. Sexual behavior problems in children can emphasize vulnerabilities in parent–child relationships or can cause them to emerge. But no matter what the preexisting state of a parent–child relationship (or sibling relationship) may be, it is important to address the relationship's foundation so that it can withstand the stress, to find areas for growth, and to support the parental figures in providing the necessary anchor for the child's emotional and psychological health.

After years of research in the field of attachment, neuroscience, successful parenting, and healthy family functioning, researchers have arrived at some basic tenets that prove useful for parents in establishing, repairing, or enhancing parent–child relationships. These basic tenets should be shared with parents throughout their treatment, in nonclinical language.

Encouraging Role Modeling and Co-Regulation

Another early topic for discussion with parents or other primary caregivers involves their affective language and expression—that is, how they talk about and express their feelings. Perhaps no other area requires such early and sustained education for children as this one. Children must learn in childhood how to identify their feelings, communicate to others how they feel, and express their feelings in socially acceptable ways. In fact, how children learn to manage their emotions is the topic of many books and a major contributor to successful child development.

There are many possible questions about emotions, and many possible suggestions. Some beliefs about and responses to emotions are gender-based: Little girls may be held and comforted when they cry, but boys may be told to "knock it off." Others are age-based: A young infant crying on an airplane trip, although painful to hear, may not elicit judgmental responses; a 7-year-old who has a temper tantrum in the grocery store may elicit much more negative reactions from others. Parents/caregivers can be helped to examine these beliefs and responses and to consider whether reworking some of them may be helpful.

Adults are often plagued with confusion about crying (both their own and their children's). A businesswoman may feel angry at herself for crying in a meeting, because she is afraid that crying will be perceived as a weakness. A businessman who cries may also feel subjected to ridicule by peers. We all seem very affected when someone cries on television during an interview. It seems that obvious shows of emotion can elicit both positive and negative responses, and they are always topics of discussion and reaction.

An important aspect of therapy is for caregivers to feel equipped to handle their own and their children's emotions. Adults can make a great contribution by helping their children learn how to negotiate and manage their emotions, both in private and in public.

SUMMARY

The research regarding the treatment of children with sexual behavior problems and their families clearly gives us much room for optimism, as both short- and long-term treatment interventions have shown positive results. It is evident from this research that young children require parents' or other primary caregivers' full engagement and willingness to provide a positive, reparative structure, along with supervision of their children in order to provide external controls. Consensus has been reached on the following three areas for treatment: (1) therapeutic attention to trauma when appropriate (i.e., a flexible approach to integration of trauma-focused treatment with interventions focused directly on sexual behavior problems); (2) active, direct caregiver involvement in treatment; and (3) inclusion of psychoeducation and CBT-focused interventions for direct management of the sexual behavior problems. Although psychoeducation and parenting programs can and should be incorporated into clinical interventions, psychoeducation topics are varied, and parenting models are ample. We have presented our own overview of work with parents/caregivers in the second part of this chapter.

Clinicians working with sexual behavior problems in children should stay aware of the research; be willing to incorporate new ways of engaging and eliciting the full cooperation of young children; and always remain cognizant of the need to join with parents/caregivers who may feel and express a wide range of intense emotions. In particular, engaging caregivers to make a full commitment to their children's therapy appears to be one of the most important clinical tasks, since parental cooperation and participation are directly related to positive treatment outcome.

Guidelines for Responding to Sexual Behavior Problems in Children

WHAT ARE SEXUAL BEHAVIOR PROBLEMS?

Sexual behavior problems vary among children. Some children may touch themselves or rub their genitals in front of others and in public places; others may show their private parts to others. Some children develop problems with language (such as talking frequently about explicit sexual acts). Some children paint inappropriate drawings of naked people, representing sexual activity in great detail. Other children convince others to take off their clothes, invite them to hide under covers, and explore their bodies. Children can even behave aggressively or in a manipulative way with other children, or give them gifts or money to let them see or touch their genitals. Some children learn to dance in a sensual or provocative way to call others' attention to them or show interest in special kinds of dances or sexy clothes. Any or all of those behaviors can occur one or more times. If these become persistent or appear to replace other, more common interests, they may be more serious sexual behavior problems.

WHAT ARE GOOD WAYS TO RESPOND TO SEXUAL BEHAVIOR PROBLEMS?

Sexual behavior problems need prompt and consistent responses by all parents and other caregivers! They also require caregivers to provide constant supervision, correction, and redirection. Responses to children's sexual behavior problems are best when they are calm and firm, sending the message that these behaviors are not appropriate and will not be ignored. The following guidelines may be helpful for parents/caregivers of children with sexual behavior problems. All caregivers are encouraged to be patient, persistent, and consistent.

Consistent and Constant Supervision

Children must be supervised at all times. Until sexual preoccupations and behavior problems decrease, children's peer play must be supervised *by adults* at all times. In addition, it is prudent to avoid sleepovers at friends' houses, and supervision must be 24/7 until children's internal controls are once again working. It's important that children know that this extra supervision is intended to help them stay safe and to help them learn to stop their behavior problems.

Friends

When children have sexual behavior problems, it is important to monitor which peers they are spending time with, because some friends might get them excited, agitated, and less likely to exhibit self-control. It is best to limit children's contact with friends with whom sexual behavior problems have already occurred.

Bathroom Use

Children need to go to the bathroom by themselves both in school and at home. It is important for them to know that personal hygiene and bathroom use are private activities and must occur in private. Any opportunity to reinforce the "privacy message" is helpful (such as when parents and children use public restrooms).

Nudity

If and when children appear nude, they must be taken to their rooms and helped to clothe themselves. Adults need to monitor children as they are coming in and out of showers or baths; sometimes children use these opportunities to "flash" others. Although this kind of family exposure can be normative, it's important to respond firmly while children are learning to use good boundaries and maintain physical privacy.

Television

Watching television is a common activity for children. However, it's important for parents and other caregivers to monitor what their children are watching. There are far too many sexually explicit or provocative shows on television. Music videos, prime-time television, soap operas, and other TV shows may contain sexually suggestive material. Since sexually aggressive children are already feeling overstimulated, this is a good time to limit their TV watching or to supervise what they watch. *Special caution:* Some parents forget that watching scary or violent movies can also get kids overly stimulated and/or agitated. It's best if children don't watch horror or violence on TV either. Needless to say, going to the movies and finding movies without sex or violence can be challenging!

Computers, Periodicals, and Other Media

If children are old enough to use computers, adults need to make sure that they are not getting into websites that have pictures of sex and violence. Parents/caregivers should try to supervise children's computer use and should be aware of the particular dangers inherent in chat rooms and social networking sites. Comic books and magazines should be examined as well. Sometimes it's surprising what children can get their hands on. Again, some of these are normative childhood activities, and children's reading and use of the Internet should be supported as long as they are not accessing inappropriate or overstimulating sexual and violent material.

Correction of Sexual Behavior Problems

It is important to address children's sexual behavior problems *each and every time* adults see them occur. When children touch themselves in public, touch or rub up against other children, use inappropriate language, make rude gestures or "sexy" movements, reenact sexual behaviors with dolls, or do anything else that seems related to sexual behavior problems, parents/caregivers should do the following:

93

- Stop them.
- Ask to speak to them in private (if they're old enough). If they are younger, correct their behavior the way you would any other behavior problem: Stop it, set limits, and give them something else to do.
- Repeat the same message: "Touching private parts is not OK. It's not OK for anyone to touch your private parts, and it's not OK for you to touch anyone else's. What you did just now [describe the behavior—for example, "asking Jimmy to suck your pee-pee"] is not okay. These behaviors have to stop." The younger the child, the fewer words you use.
- Set the consequence (something you've already spoken about).
- Keep this simple. Speak in a calm voice. You might want to take a little time so you can calm down. (If you do take time, have the child wait in a safe place.)

Redirection

After parents/caregivers correct the sexual behavior problems and set consequences, they should be sure to talk to children about what the children *can* do. They might want to make a list of behaviors that children can engage in with friends or siblings, under supervision. They might also want to practice or role-play appropriate greetings or other expressions of affection or playfulness.

Family Talks

It's important to recognize that most children who have sexual behavior problems are trying to show thoughts or feelings that might be worrisome or confusing to them. Some children who develop sexual behavior problems have been physically or sexually abused themselves; in these cases, they have difficulty with unwanted thoughts and feelings regarding their abuse. Sometimes their sexual behavior problems seem to "pop up" out of nowhere. At other times, certain situations or people may remind these children of their abuse, and this remembering can cause problematic thoughts, feelings, or sensations. In order to be helpful to such children, as well as to children with sexual behavior problems who have no abuse history, parents and other caregivers are encouraged to be consistent and clear in setting firm and immediate limits and consequences. Parents/caregivers also need to redirect their children to other fun activities, and they need to teach them how to express difficult feelings.

Children can also benefit from hearing positive messages from parents and other caregivers about sexuality. Adults might want to develop some statements that are comfortable for them to say with conviction—for example, "Sex is something that grownups do to show their love for each other." If children who have been abused are older and seem to be having confusion about their sexuality, adults can help them differentiate between sexual abuse and making love.

In addition, there are some basic messages that most families provide to young children:

- "Your body belongs to you. Your body has lots of parts, including your private parts." (It can be fun to have kids list their body parts and then define which ones are *private*. For example, "Private parts are the ones we cover up with our bathing suits when we go swimming.")
- "Private parts are called private because you keep them private. You don't show them to other people, and you don't touch other peoples' privates."
- "It's not OK for anyone to touch children's private parts unless parents are trying to keep their children clean when they are babies, or when nurses or doctors are trying to keep children healthy. Doctors and nurses might need to look at private parts or put medicine on them."
- Parents/other caregivers may feel more or less comfortable talking about children touching their own privates. Most caregivers feel comfortable saying that it's OK for children to touch their privates as long as they do it in private. Caregivers must develop the messages and values they want to transmit to their children.

Finally, and *most importantly:*

- Sometimes when children are touched on their private parts, they are told to keep it secret. Keeping such secrets can make children feel worried, guilty, ashamed, confused, angry, or sad. Children should be reminded that if someone tells them to keep a secret from their parents or caregivers, that's a good sign that the secret must be told.

WHAT ARE OTHER WAYS PARENTS/CAREGIVERS
CAN HELP THEIR CHILDREN?

Children need to be told what they do well, and they need small rewards for accomplishing goals. Sometimes parents/caregivers get distracted by supervising children and making sure they don't do something wrong or inappropriate. It's important to *catch them being good or doing well*.

Building self-esteem is a slow process. It's almost like using building blocks to make a tall structure: The stronger (wider, sturdier) the foundation, the easier the structure will stay up. Parents and other caregivers can make a big contribution to children's self-esteem by finding positive things to say to the children each day.

Trust also builds slowly. Children will trust adults as soon as they can. This cannot be rushed. The best advice for parents and other caregivers is to take every opportunity to show that they are trustworthy (that is, that they will follow through on their promises to children).

Children should be encouraged to play well with others. When children play, they hardly notice that they are being supervised.

Role modeling is very important as well. The old adage "Do as I do, not as I say," is mostly true. Most children learn from the adults around them. Parents/caregivers need to take opportunities to teach children some important lessons through their own behavior, such as how to express emotions safely and calmly, how to be respectful of others, and how to ask others for things. Adults also have many opportunities to model behaviors relating to privacy, boundaries, physical affection, and so forth.

If children are in therapy for their behavioral problems, parents/caregivers must be sure to stay in close contact with the children's therapists, jot down any questions, and make sure that they feel comfortable asking the therapists whatever they need to ask.

CHILDREN'S SUPERVISION IN SCHOOL

Finally, parents/caregivers of children with sexual behavior problems have to decide how to inform the school about their children's problems. This could be of benefit to avoid problems if such a child is without supervision in the company of other children. Many schools have rules that children should go in pairs to the bathroom. This practice could pose a risk if a child has sexual

behavior problems. The parents/caregivers need to decide how much information they are going to share. Sometimes they can only say that a child is having
problems with limits in personal space and needs supervision when he or she
is with others.

Thank you so much for reading this, and please feel free to ask questions
if something is not clear or if something needs to be added. Your thoughts and
questions are always welcome.

I, _____, have read and discussed this
information, and I have had the opportunity to ask questions, determine the
plan of action, and obtain orientation. I agree to work on the sexual behavior
problems with my child.

_____   _____

Name   Date

_____   _____

Name   Date

FORM 5.2

Affective Scaling Worksheet

Choose one or more feelings, and then circle the size of each feeling.

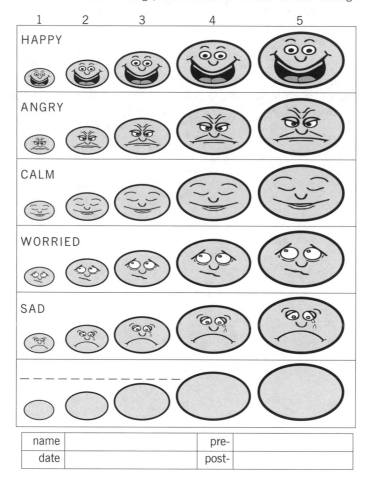

name		pre-	
date		post-	

FORM 5.3 Body Thermometer

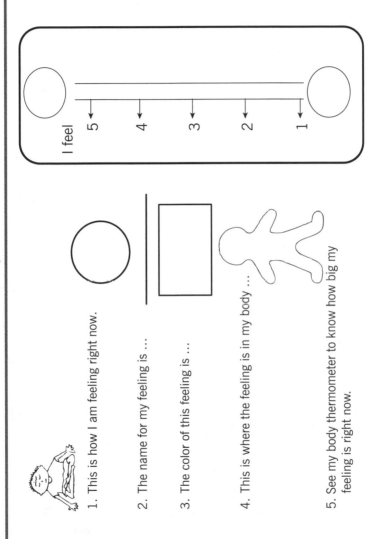

1. This is how I am feeling right now.

2. The name for my feeling is …

3. The color of this feeling is …

4. This is where the feeling is in my body …

5. See my body thermometer to know how big my feeling is right now.

I feel

5

4

3

2

1

CHAPTER SIX

The Boundary Project Model

This chapter provides information about a therapy model that is research-informed, practical, and family-friendly. The program has been implemented in several settings over the last two decades; it has evolved into a structured, manualized approach that enjoys good treatment outcomes as indicated by both parent and child reports, and more recently by pre- and posttreatment testing of specific target behaviors. The Boundary Project is an integrative, family-focused model for children ages 4–11 with sexual behavior problems (and their parents or other primary caregivers). The model encompasses basic principles of trauma-focused therapy and includes a range of other approaches, including CBT, expressive therapies (play, sand, and art), psychoeducation, attachment-based techniques, and relaxation exercises (e.g., guided relaxation, breathing, mindfulness). These strategies are designed to advance the goals of reducing sexual behavior problems while addressing underlying factors in both children and their families.

SPECIAL FEATURES OF THE BOUNDARY PROJECT

The Boundary Project model is family-focused (i.e., it requires equal treatment investment from a child and at least one consistent caregiver). Treatment goals can be delivered in individual, group, and family therapy modalities.

The Boundary Project is a phase-based treatment model loosely based on Judith Herman's (1992) three phases of treatment: safety and relationship building; addressing traumatic material; and affiliation and future orientation. Obviously, additional attention during the middle phase of treatment is given to addressing the sexual behavior problems in the context of identified past traumatic events, as well as to the potentially traumatic impact of environmental variables or family dynamics. In our opinion, identifying the underlying causes of sexual behavior problems, and setting clear and consistent limits, must be done within the context of helping children process whatever past traumas ignite or fuel their current behaviors. Many children who have been abused, and have not had opportunities to process their abuse, may utilize abusive behaviors in an effort to work through their pain and emotional distress, confusions, or worries. In addition, significant clinical attention is paid to enhancing parent–child relationships, so that parents/caregivers can feel adequate and confident to provide support and guidance to their children. We have noted that as the adults' confidence increases, their children's perceptions of them may become more positive. That is, the children may be able to view these adults as sources of nurturing and consistent care, and may start to welcome limit setting and rewards. Thus work with caregivers of children who have sexual behavior problems must identify and incorporate family strengths; must provide the caregivers with clear guidance about effective parenting approaches; and must help them develop their own coping and self-care strategies, so that their empathic and consistent abilities are maximized and their fears, doubts, and worries are decreased.

Finally, the Boundary Project is unique in that it values, allows, encourages, and invites expressive therapies and utilizes child-centered play therapy in recognition of children's ability and willingness to play out their difficulties through posttraumatic play (Gil, 2010b). The Boundary Project advances trauma-focused goals by utilizing such approaches, which provide children with broad opportunities to engage and invest in the treatment process. Expressive therapies, including play and art (Sobol & Schneider, 1998), are woven into treatment interventions not only to enhance the potential for affective expression, but to provide opportunities to process difficult clinical material through introspection, insight, and compensatory externalized activities. Strategies from evidence-based programs, such as trauma-focused CBT, are incorporated as children become better able to regulate, attend, and utilize cognitive processes. Perry (2009) emphasizes sequencing treatment so that interventions are sensitive to changes in children's brain functioning. As an example, a child who is impulsive, defiant, and dysregulated may not be able to engage in cognitive reflecting and processing. It will be better to deal with the child's dysregulation first through activities such as guided relaxation, breathing, and positive/empathic (nurturing) responses, before introducing discussions that require the child's cortex to be functioning age-appropriately. These simple principles about the child's developing brain are woven into parental education about how to respond to children's behaviors and what types of responses may have the most positive outcomes. Siegel and Payne Bryson (2011) present very useful strategies for keeping in mind the "whole brain" of a child.

TREATMENT FORMATS

Children's sexual behavior problems are assessed via the structured ASBPC process described in Chapter Four, which respects children's developmental ages and levels of functioning so that they (and their families) can be placed on the appropriate treatment track. Groups are usually divided by children's age ranges (4–6, 7–9, and 9–11 years). All groups require consistent parent/caregiver participation throughout the 12-week process. For the most part, caregivers' participation has not been an issue in the Boundary Project, for several reasons: Their attendance can be mandated by protective service agencies; someone has to bring young children to therapy (as opposed to adolescents, who can sometimes get themselves to therapy on their own); and caregivers are often strongly invested in ameliorating their children's sexual behavior problems, and recognize that they need and want guidance in the best ways of responding to their children.

Individual therapy is recommended if a group setting is not determined to be appropriate for a particular child or presenting problem, or if there is a waiting period for a new group to start and a family's treatment needs are compelling. In those cases, treatment principles are presented and processed in an individual setting, and will be repeated if the same child is considered a candidate for a group following individual treatment. That is, the same target concepts will be reinforced in a peer group, where there are opportunities for role play and destigmatization.

Finally, there are some cases that truly benefit from whole-family therapy sessions because the family members seem to function better with individualized attention than with participation in groups. Some parents/caregivers do not "fit" well into groups for a variety of reasons (difficulty with processing information, problematic communication style, profound histories of past trauma, developmental delays, need for diverse languages). Children may have difficulties integrating into groups for these and other reasons—most often their dysregulated behaviors and their inability to control themselves, due to the apparent hyperarousal or agitation of being with others. Thus being able to provide children and families with help in a variety of formats is crucial for their and the program's success.

TREATMENT PHASES AND GOALS

Treatment is initiated following the assessment, which, as described in Chapter Four, seeks to ascertain the child's overall functioning; further determine the depth and scope of the problem behaviors; and gather impressions of etiological and maintaining factors. The assessment allows the clinician to prioritize treatment objectives and informs the direct management of identified or suspected sexual behavior problems—including safety and supervision considerations (and any immediate measures that need to be taken to ensure the safety of other children while the referred child is in treatment).

Based on current, research-informed knowledge regarding sexual behavior problems in young children (see Chapters One and Five), the treatment foci include the following:

1. Developing a relational foundation with children and their parents/caregivers.
2. Encouraging the identification and appropriate expression of affect in both children and adults.
3. Correcting cognitive distortions about sexual behavior problems and their impact.
4. Addressing histories of past abuse or current high-risk factors.
5. Increasing the children's and families' awareness of underlying causes of the problem behaviors.
6. Encouraging improved social interactions and boundaries, as well as appropriate use of resources.

PARENTAL/CAREGIVER GROUPS
AND INTEGRATION OF EDUCATION

While child clients attend a 12-week structured group, parents/caregivers meet in an adjacent room, learning and practicing many of the same target concepts as their children. In the last 25–30 minutes of the concurrent groups, adults and children join together so that they can tell each other what they learned in their respective sessions. This gives clinicians an opportunity to observe parent–child interactions, encourage open communication, and offer correction when lessons appear to be misunderstood or misarticulated. When a child is in the 12-week *individual* therapy process, parents/caregivers join the session for the last 15 minutes for a review of what the child has learned in his or her therapy session. Once Boundary Project treatment is completed, caregivers and children may be provided with additional services that may include additional individual or family therapy.

Family therapy sessions are provided in order to review psychoeducational materials, assess family strengths and vulnerabilities, ensure caregiver supervision, and assist in the process of restoring trust while providing external controls.

ACTIVITIES FOR TRANSITIONS IN/OUT OF SESSIONS

Structure, routine, and consistency are important factors for all young children, and particularly important for children who are referred for treatment because of a traumatic experience and/or serious behavioral problems. Children are more likely to ease into challenging activities if they have time to make the transition in and out of therapy sessions in ways that promote self-awareness and relaxation.

Affective Scaling (Self-Awareness)

Affective scaling activities are introduced at the beginning of each session ("check-in") and again at the end of each session ("check-out"). The specific goals for affective scaling twice per session are to encourage children to identify and acknowledge their feelings; to assist them in determining the intensity of their feelings; and to help them learn ways to increase or decrease the intensity of their feelings. Helping children build emotional language, express emotions in appropriate ways, and learn to understand their emotional needs are important aspects of any therapy with children (Jaffe & Gardner, 2006; Gottman, 1997).

The Affective Scaling Worksheet and the Body Thermometer (see Forms 5.2 and 5.3 at the end of Chapter Five) allow children to engage in affective self-monitoring at the beginning and end of each treatment session, in either individual or group therapy formats. Once children point to the feeling state drawn on the Body Thermometer, clinicians show them the Affective Scaling Worksheet, where the selected feeling is provided in five sizes (from small to large). Then clinicians ask children to "point to the size of the feeling that you're feeling right now." For the most part, we have seen positive effects of treatment sessions, in that negative feelings decrease and positive feelings increase; however, on occasion, children indicate the reverse (i.e., positive feelings turn negative, sometimes due to difficult topics or not wanting to leave).

Children are asked to make a drawing of any new feeling face that they believe is missing from the Affective Scaling Worksheet and that they need to include. In addition, it is important for children to know that people often have more than one feeling at the same time.

Parents/caregivers are encouraged to reinforce affective scaling at home by "checking in" on how their children are feeling before and after everyday activities, at the beginning and at the end of the day, and before and after unusual or distressing events. These adults are also encouraged to model the use of affective scaling by naming and scaling their own emotions throughout the day (e.g., "Mommy's proud feeling is a 5, because you came home and did your homework without me telling you to," or "Daddy's happy feeling is a 2, because I'm stuck in traffic, and I feel my frustrated feeling growing from a 3 to a 4!"). Children and caregivers are encouraged to notice any changes in feelings and in the intensity of those feelings, and to reflect on what may have created these shifts in feeling states. This will begin to bring their awareness to ways in which their thoughts, feelings, and actions are interconnected and can be redirected and managed.

Clinicians are also advised to keep a set of "feeling cards" available, so that children can point to additional feelings that might better capture their emotional states.

Relaxation Exercises

A relaxation exercise (controlled breathing, progressive muscle relaxation, guided visualization, mindfulness meditation, etc.) is also provided at both the beginning and end of each session, to orient parents/caregivers and children to therapy hour. The specific goals for relaxation exercises are to help both children and adults sharpen and ready their minds for active learning; to train children to stay calm and centered with sustained attention; and, as noted above, to help children and adults make the transition in and out of therapy sessions (Greco &

Hayes, 2008; Hawn, 2011).* The Boundary Project incorporates a 3- to 5-minute relaxation exercise immediately following the affective scaling "check-in." A second relaxation exercise follows the session-specific lesson or activity (just prior to the affective scaling "check-out"). Mindfulness and relaxation exercises can be used in either individual therapy, parent–child dyads, or group therapy.

Parents/caregivers are again encouraged to promote mindfulness and relaxation at home by using relaxation materials with a guided meditation component. (A new iTunes app called Breathe2Relax is user-friendly to children.)

TREATMENT OBJECTIVES:
THE LESSONS OF THE BOUNDARY PROJECT

The Boundary Project has 12 primary treatment objectives. These are summarized for children and caregivers in Form 6.1.

1. Safety review and setting the context.
2. Defining physical and emotional boundaries.
3. Affective tension: Identification, scaling, and safe expression of affect.
4. Differentiating and understanding types of touches.
5. Identifying the origins of the "touching problem."
6. Learning the "cognitive triangle": Connecting thoughts to feelings to actions.
7. Impulse control: The brain and the touching problem.
8. Externalizing and containing the problem.
9. Personal mastery and self-esteem building.
10. Identifying resources/supports and asking for help.
11. Reinforcement: Lesson review and preparation for discharge.
12. Safety review and goodbye celebration.

Next, we provide a brief review of these 12 objectives.

Safety Review and Setting the Context

Session 1 sets the context for why children are in therapy and what will happen. Clinicians explain openly that the children have been

---

* To learn about scientific research that has provided evidence for the positive effects of mindfulness, go to this website (*www.thehawnfoundation.org/research*).

referred because of sexual behavior problems, and that when they come to therapy clinicians will talk with them about ways to stop the problem behaviors. The goals of this session are to introduce children to each other (in group treatment) and to the physical environment; to establish rules or guidelines for children's behaviors during sessions; to introduce and define key terms; and to establish and practice beginning and ending rituals (affect identification, affective scaling, and relaxation).

Defining Physical and Emotional Boundaries

The goals of Session 2 are to assess children's current understanding of boundaries and physical space; to define the term "boundaries," in both physical and emotional senses; and to review and practice recognizing and respecting each other's limits and boundaries during the session (Gil & Shaw, 2010; Cook, 2007).

Affective Tension: Identification, Scaling, and Safe Expression of Affect

Goals for Session 3 are to improve affect identification and regulation; to continue with affective scaling, and to introduce tools for safe expression of feelings; to identify affective states "in the moment" and introduce the concept of intensity; and to lay the foundation for integrating methods for reducing body tension and responding appropriately to the "touching idea/feeling/problem."

Differentiating and Understanding Types of Touches

Goals of Session 4 are to help children recognize different kinds of touches and how they feel different from one another; to categorize types of touches; and to begin the process of working explicitly to stop inappropriate and problematic touches by group members. The Three Types of Touches curriculum (Pennsylvania Coalition Against Rape, n.d.) may prove useful in this session.

Identifying the Origins of the "Touching Problem"

The goals for Session 5 are to acknowledge that the "touching idea" grew into a "touching problem" behavior for each child in the room; to identify the origins of the idea and to brainstorm ways the problem grew to where it is currently; to identify child- or family-specific factors that contributed to its growth; and to illustrate that a problem can both grow and shrink.

Learning the "Cognitive Triangle"

The goals for Session 6 are to show children the relationship among what they think, what they feel, and what they do; to explain the concept of the "cognitive triangle," with examples of how the three elements interact; to introduce the concept of "cognitive distortions" or "thinking problems," as well as thought substitution; and to create a foundation for exploring how this information can be used with the touching problem (Narelle, 2011; Stallard, 2002; Lamb-Shapiro, 2000).

Impulse Control: The Brain and the Touching Problem

The goals of Session 7 are to introduce the concept of impulses and urges originating from the brain; to introduce the concept of controlling responses, regardless of the type or intensity of an impulse (i.e., non-sexual and sexual thoughts and feelings do not have to result in action); to provide education on thought stopping/thought interruption; and to demonstrate the effectiveness of relaxation and mindfulness/meditation in reducing tense feelings and, alternatively, in problem solving.

Externalizing and Containing the Problem

Goals for Session 8 are to explore children's thoughts, feelings, and perceptions of themselves as these are related to each child's problem behaviors; to give children opportunities to use their projective abilities to externalize the behavior and examine the problem from a safe enough distance; to promote children's awareness that the problem can be made smaller and contained; and to emphasize the existence of resources and helpers to keep the problem controlled.

Personal Mastery and Self-Esteem Building

The goals for Session 9 are to identify and celebrate children's internal and external resources; to promote personal control over feelings and actions; and to increase children's self-esteem (specifically, by helping them to see their problem behaviors as separate from their own sense of self).

Identifying Resources/Supports and Asking for Help

The goals of Session 10 are to encourage children to focus on the safe and appropriate people who serve as resources to them in their lives, and to provide opportunities for children and parents to identify and share their collective family resources and supports.

Reinforcement: Lesson Review and Preparing for Discharge

The goals of Session 11 are to review and reinforce core concepts; to provide parents/caregivers with support and clarify their questions or concerns; and to prepare for the ending of treatment and the transfer of learning to the home environment.

Safety Review and Goodbye Celebration

The goals of Session 12 are to celebrate the completion of the treatment process; to review all lessons and discussions; to review children's art products; to encourage a discussion of the importance of saying good-bye; to help children remember the treatment (and, in group treatment, the group members) by taking mental pictures; and to give each child a small gift and a certificate of completion.

These treatment objectives are introduced and reiterated in 12 structured once-weekly sessions, and are reinforced by parents/caregivers through child-friendly and solution-focused activities. As mentioned earlier, depending on treatment needs identified through the assessment process, these 12 sessions can be conducted in individual, group, or family therapy formats.

CHALLENGES AND RESPONSES

The Boundary Project model is designed to ameliorate sexual behavior problems in young children while addressing the familial and environmental factors that may underlie, maintain, or exacerbate those behaviors. Based on current research, Boundary Project interventions target two primary levels: (1) treatment, education, and supervision of the children's sexual behavior problems; and (2) promoting parent–child relationships through requiring active participation by caregivers in session and at home (at-home relationship-building activities).

The ultimate aims of this program include the following:

- To create an environment of safety, trust, and comfort.
- To address the safety needs of other children in the referred children's homes, schools, and communities.
- To replace maladaptive coping strategies with healthy and helpful strategies.
- To increase external monitoring across settings.
- To help the children develop internal controls.
- To reduce sexual behavior problems.
- To reduce factors that contributed to the development of the sexual behavior problems.
- To teach and engage caregivers in appropriate ways to respond to and supervise children.
- To provide psychoeducation, support, and resources to caregivers.

Working with young children who have sexual behavior problems has special challenges, which have been identified in earlier chapters. Through trial and error, we have learned the importance of ensuring that clinical approaches are structured, developmentally appropriate, engaging, time-sensitive, and repetitive. In addition, treatment sessions that engage the "whole child" by including intellectual, emotional, physical, and expressive activities have greater potential to elicit more enthusiastic and whole-hearted participation. Moreover, as suggested by current research, caregivers' cooperation and involvement are pivotal to short-term treatment effectiveness, as well as to long-term recovery from those factors that underlie the behaviors.

Through the implementation of this model, we have found that certain approaches and activities greatly enhance the potential for successful treatment. For example, a treatment structure that includes time-limited "lessons" is important, given children's limited attention span (the lessons last for no longer than 20 minutes each session). In addition, we have found it useful to ensure that parents/caregivers are receiving concurrent psychoeducational interventions, so that they know and can reinforce what their children are learning. We have also found that frequent and repeated reviews of material within each session can be very useful before new concepts are introduced. Throughout our treatment, we reiterate what lessons have been learned before we move on to a new concept. Finally, we find it imperative both to demonstrate and to have children and caregivers practice activities so that they can be repeated at home; it is not sufficient simply to give verbal directives. Clinical demonstration and practice are critical strategies in ensuring success.

Finally, we have found that parents/caregivers and children benefit greatly from the focus on identifying affective states and levels, as well as from learning breathing and mindfulness exercises. One aspect of our interventions that was changed, based on family feedback, was the incorporation of family relaxation strategies in place of individual ones Families reported that they benefited from doing the relaxation strategies together, and both children and adults found them easier to request of each other and repeat together once they practiced doing them in the clinical setting.

GAUGING PROGRESS OBJECTIVELY

Clinicians are strongly encouraged to incorporate pre- and posttreatment measurements of functioning as a way to evaluate their work. The use of a simple pre- and posttreatment design that establishes a baseline of concerns and assesses those concerns after treatment can be very beneficial. Standardized measures administered at the start and end of treatment can be used not only to inform clinicians about the success of treatment, but to guide decision making about a child's and family's treatment needs after discharge from the structured phase of treatment; the results of these measures can then be incorporated into feedback sessions with caregivers and/or referring agencies. Clinicians are encouraged to administer the following child and parent report measures (most of which have been mentioned in Chapter Four) at the time of intake and again at the close of the treatment program: the Trauma Symptom Checklist for Children (TSCC) or Trauma Symptom Checklist for Young Children (TSCYC) (Briere, 1996, 2005); the appropriate version of the Child Behavior Checklist (CBCL) for a child's age (Achenbach & Rescorla, 2000, 2001); the Child Sexual Behavior Inventory (CSBI; Friedrich, 1997); and the Parent–Child Relationship Inventory (PCRI; Gerard, 1994). Results can be used to make posttreatment therapy recommendations and to convey safety considerations for home, school, and community supports and supervisors.

In addition, play- and art-based activities can be incorporated into the evaluation of treatment, as well as periods of child-centered play therapy (see Chapter Four). Children's expressive art products should be carefully reviewed to gain increased insight into children's perceptions of self and others. In addition, many of these externalized products provide opportunities for children to externalize their worries symbolically, reflect, and manage their affect gradually, in what Gil (2012) calls children's natural and self-selected gradual exposure. These opportunities should be evaluated as well.

SUMMARY

The Boundary Project is a structured, family-based program designed to focus on children's sexual behavior problems, engage parents/caregivers as external controls, and encourage children to understand and explore the emotional states that usually fuel their acting-out behaviors. Boundary Project staff members provide children with consistent, empathic, and repetitive role modeling and redirection, so that children develop a sense of mastery and control over inappropriate behaviors. In addition, because the caregivers are active participants in helping their children and reviewing and modeling lessons learned in treatment, a more consistent transfer of learning can occur.

Parents/caregivers are given empathic understanding themselves, and their frustrations and fears are addressed consistently. In our experience, these adults may be hesitant when first referred to the Boundary Project; may feel stressed out about having to manage their difficult schedules and/or openly discuss private matters; and may come to treatment feeling guilty or inadequate to solve their problems. Parental groups are support groups as well as opportunities for psychoeducation, and in our experience caregivers will participate more fully if they feel that their basic fears and frustrations are understood and explored. Clinical tasks for parents/caregivers are listed elsewhere (see Chapter Five), but it is important to state that adults' attendance and cooperation are good predictors of children's treatment success and amelioration of sexual behavior problems.

The group treatment version of the Boundary Project proposes collateral groups for parents/caregivers and children, which are brought together to reinforce lessons, to promote functional parent–child interactions, and to model open communication about behaviors that might have been kept secret in the past. Therapy is demystified by having children share with their caregivers the steps in their recovery process. In addition, family members are encouraged to participate actively in becoming comfortable with the use of suggested techniques throughout the week between sessions.

A unique aspect of our program is that children can receive the intervention in individual, group, or family therapy settings, and can even go through two cycles if clinical decisions dictate. In addition, the interventions are infused with playful, physical, holistic learning approaches that take into consideration the developmental needs of children and their families, as well as gender differences in children and the uniqueness of each child. Clinical staff members are patient, nonjudgmental, and kind, and possess a repertoire of ways to introduce and implement lesson plans.

In short, the Boundary Project is an integrated, research-informed model that incorporates the latest data on the subject; engages children with expressive techniques; incorporates valuable principles of trauma-focused CBT; teaches children to understand their minds and bodies; and engages parents or other primary caregivers as empathic, firm, and dependable limit setters and nurturing guides to their children.

FORM 6.1 Boundary Project Treatment: 12-Session Treatment Objectives for Children and Caregivers

My parent and I meet separately, yet we do four things the same each session...

Point to how I feel...	then... choose a size for my feeling.	Relax my body	Show my parent what I learned...
(or choose my very own feeling!)	*(to show how BIG or small it feels)*	and focus my mind	*(and see what my parent learned!)*

My parent and I will learn and practice new skills together

1. Introductions and Safety Safety review, session structure, and getting to know each other	**2. What Is a Boundary?** Defining physical and emotional boundaries and how they make us feel	**3. Coping with Tension** Rating our feelings... and safe expression of BIG feelings	**4. Three Kinds of Touches** Learn and discuss loving, "ouch," and "uh-oh" touches
5. Why Did the Problem Start and How Did It Grow? Looking at the Roots of the Problem	**6. Learning the CBT Triangle** Thoughts – Feelings – Actions	**7. Impulse Control** My Brain and the Touching Problem	**8. Taking a Look Inside** Externalizing and shrinking the problem as a family
9. Personal Mastery Self-esteem building: Identifying my superhero powers!	**10. Identifying My Resources** Supports and asking for help	**11. Lesson Review** REVIEW Review and family safety planning	**12. Safety Review** Goodbye celebration and graduation

CHAPTER SEVEN

The Case of Kayla

REFERRAL INFORMATION

Kayla B, an 8-year-old girl, was referred for specialized treatment of sexual behavior problems by a local child protective services worker. The referral followed Kayla's second suspension from school for repeated inappropriate and, more recently, aggressive sexual behaviors. Before treatment was initiated, an assessment was conducted to gain insight into the origin, type, and extent of the sexual behavior problems, as well as into the parents' and the school's responses to date. The referring incident occurred on a school bus where Kayla grabbed a 6-year-old boy's penis, then asked him to touch her "down there" (while she grabbed the younger child's hand and placed his hand under her pants and underwear). Kayla had a history of intimidating and bullying younger children on the school bus and playground; true to form, she told this child that she would hurt him and "tell your mom and the bus driver that *you* started the game" if he did not comply or told anyone. In spite of feeling afraid, the young boy told his mother about Kayla's behavior when he got home, and the incident was reported to the school.

The school guidance counselor contacted child protective services, as required by law, to assert the school's concerns about Kayla's sexually abusive behaviors. Kayla was also suspended, pending the completion of a "school threat assessment." The referring social worker commented that the school personnel suspected Kayla was being sexually abused. Following this most recent incident, the school viewed Kayla as "sexually aggressive" and a risk to other children. The principal told

Kayla's parents that any subsequent incidents would result in expulsion, as well as an immediate referral to an alternative or specialized learning environment. Home-bound educational services were being actively explored at the time of the referral to our clinic. The local child protective services worker contacted Kayla's mother and stepfather and conducted interviews with them, with Kayla, and with Kayla's siblings. No disclosures of parental abuse were made by Kayla or her siblings. Given Kayla's escalating sexual behaviors, however, the safety of the two younger children was listed as a current concern, and the child protective services worker informed Kayla's parents that she could not be around her siblings unsupervised.

PSYCHOSOCIAL BACKGROUND

Kayla was the oldest of three children and was in the second grade at the time of the assessment. She was the only child born of her mother and biological father. Kayla's mother was European American and her father was African American. Kayla had intermittent contact with her father, who now resided in another state; contact was limited to holidays and occasions when he might be in town. Kayla's mother and father had never married, and Kayla had been raised by her stepfather since the age of 3½ years. At the time of referral, Kayla's half-sister (Katie) was 3 years of age, and her half-brother (Kaleb) was 2 years of age. According to Mrs. B, Kayla frequently said that she was going to run away and live with her father.

Mrs. B stated that Kayla's prenatal development and birth history were unremarkable, other than a period of time when she had financial and emotional stress. (Kayla's father had moved out of state shortly following her birth, and there was very limited family support to the then 21-year-old single mother.) Mrs. B reported that she herself had a significant history of trauma (physical abuse); she also had symptoms of clinical depression by adolescence, and these were particularly severe during her pregnancy and throughout Kayla's infancy. Overall, Kayla's infancy and early development suggested that she was physically healthy and reached all major developmental milestones within age-expected limits. Mrs. B had been prescribed antidepressant medication but did not take it consistently, reportedly because she lacked adequate health insurance to cover costs. Neither Kayla nor her mother had ever received outpatient therapy services.

As noted above, Kayla resided at this time with her mother and step-father, who was also European American. Kayla's skin color was much darker than that of her two siblings, who were born to her mother and stepfather. During the clinical interview with Mrs. B, the mother's negative feelings about Kayla's biological father were evident and clearly not disguised in the presence of Kayla. Kayla's mother talked disparagingly about him (e.g., "He's a liar . . . he doesn't care about anyone but himself . . . he will do anything to get attention"). Kayla's mother stated twice that her daughter's behaviors were similar to her father's behaviors, adding both times, "She's just like him." Throughout the assessment, Kayla's mother appeared depressed, overwhelmed, and angry. Her frustration with Kayla's high energy was immediately and consistently expressed, as was her pessimism about Kayla's future. Her affect brightened when she talked about her two other children, but she again added negative comments about Kayla to her reporting, including "They are starting to act up because they watch Kayla do it." During Mrs. B's reporting, all negative experiences in the household or tension among family members were attributed to Kayla's personality or behaviors.

According to Mrs. B, Kayla "has always been difficult." When asked to describe "difficult," Mrs. B stated that she was demanding, manipulative, and hard to satisfy. She implied that "no one" could soothe or comfort Kayla as an infant, because she "caused problems from the day she was born."

Kayla had completed preschool and kindergarten without difficulty, and her mother reported these years as better for Kayla and the family. After the stepfather moved into the home when Kayla was 3½ years of age, her mother had the two younger children in less than 2 years. Initially Kayla enjoyed being the older sister, and her mother stated that she did well in kindergarten, including above-average academic performance. Kayla was described as "calmer" in kindergarten; she had several friends; and her teachers described her as "outgoing, bright, confident, and full of energy." She did have some difficulty with following instructions and paying attention, and could become upset quickly, but not to the degree of needing in-school intervention until the first grade.

According to Mrs. B, Kayla had a regular sleep pattern and consistent appetite. However, she added that Kayla had frequent nightmares but was usually able to go back to sleep afterward. Kayla did not seek out her mother for comfort after a nightmare, but rather asked her stepfather to bring her back to bed. Kayla was reported to have started wetting the bed approximately 18 months ago, with accidents on average twice per week. No other major medical issues or previous hospitalizations were reported.

Kayla's stepfather, Mr. B, attended each assessment appointment and was quick to defend Kayla during her mother's negative reporting. Mr. B worked two jobs outside the home and had very little daily interaction with Kayla. He described his relationship with Kayla as "OK, but it could be better." Mr. B stated that their home was often loud and chaotic; he frequently arrived home to find Mrs. B upset or yelling at Kayla, and Kayla either mad or crying after an incident with her mother. Mr. B appeared to be quiet, calm, passive, and avoidant of confrontation. He often stopped sharing his impressions when interrupted by Mrs. B.

During the intake interview, Mrs. B added that the family had current serious financial pressures and that she was 3 months pregnant. The child protective services worker described Kayla's home as untidy and the mother as clearly overwhelmed with daily tasks and the care of the two toddlers. Kayla was not involved in any extracurricular activities, although she was interested in dance, Girl Scouts, and sports. Mrs. B reported that she could not afford extra activities, but stated that she would look into this when her two youngest children were older. Kayla was home from school by 2:30 P.M. and did not go outside to play, other than riding her bike on Saturdays when her stepfather could watch her in the neighborhood.

When asked about how the parents disciplined Kayla, Mrs. B immediately stated, "Nothing works." She noted that she attempted to redirect Kayla and had tried time out, but confided that her go-to discipline methods at the moment were yelling and threats of spanking, "because that's all that works with her." Mrs. B admitted to spanking Kayla approximately once a week and often in the midst of an argument. Mr. B stated that he preferred to approach Kayla when she was calm and when the other children were already in bed. He found her reasonable and agreeable to his suggestions at these times, but he admitted that while her intentions might be good, her follow-through was not great, especially with her mother.

Regarding Kayla's sexual behaviors, her school principal and current teacher reported that they had had concerns about these behaviors since Kayla started first grade. Specific concerns included sexualized language and behavior. An incident earlier in Kayla's second-grade year had resulted in her first school suspension, and was followed by increased supervision in common areas of the school. In the previous school incident, Kayla had entered the bathroom stall of a same-age (physically smaller and reserved) female peer; locked the stall door behind herself and the other child; and then told the youngster she would be her "best friend" if she showed her private parts to Kayla. Teachers added that Kayla regularly made jokes about genitals, sang inappropriate songs, had knowledge of sexual language and acts beyond what they considered typical for her age, and had given other children drawings of sexual acts (e.g., kissing, two figures lying together on a bed with the word "sex" written as the title). When asked to describe Kayla, her current teacher used words like "savvy, smart, and energetic," as well as "loud, needy, manipulative, and sneaky." The principal added that Kayla often sought more attention from the male staff than the female staff, including "seductive dancing and gyrating" during gym class and recess. Kayla also often told others that she had "a *lot* of boyfriends" and was known to seek attention from older boys at the school during unstructured periods of the day.

ASSESSMENT PROCESS

In an effort to explore the nature and extent of Kayla's sexual behavior problems, the ASBPC process was undertaken to determine treatment needs of Kayla and her family. As described in detail in Chapter Four, this assessment model includes inviting children to do play-based assessment tasks (including art, play, and sand therapies). Another special feature of this assessment model is that it allows children to engage in nondirective, child-centered play therapy, which trained clinicians can then assess for content and process. In addition, this assessment model involves gathering collateral information (e.g., from teachers and school personnel) and taking a developmental history; reviewing school evaluations; and evaluating results from a number of standardized assessment measures, which can include the CSBI (Friedrich, 1997); the age-appropriate version of the CBCL, completed by parents or teachers (Achenbach & Rescorla, 2000, 2001); and the TSCC or TSCYC, as appropriate (Briere, 1996, 2005).

Standardized Assessment of Nonsexual Behaviors

Both Kayla's teachers and her parents had noted that she was exhibiting consistently and increasingly problematic behaviors, particularly aggression, intrusiveness, and noncompliance. Given these concerns and Kayla's other areas of difficulties, Kayla was asked to complete the TSCC—a child report measure of posttraumatic stress and related psychological symptomatology in children ages 8–16 years who have experienced traumatic events (such as physical or sexual abuse, major loss, or natural disasters) or who have witnessed violence. This 54-item measure covers a variety of domains, including anxiety, depression, anger, posttraumatic stress, dissociation, overt dissociation, fantasy, sexual concerns, sexual preoccupation, and sexual distress (Briere, 1996). According to this parent report, Kayla's scores were clinically significant in the domains of anger, anxiety, posttraumatic stress, sexual concerns, and sexual distress. The Posttraumatic Stress scale of this instrument reflects such symptoms as intrusive sensations, thoughts, memories of painful past events, nightmares, cognitive avoidance of memories and negative thoughts, and fear of women or men.

Results from the CBCL parent report (Achenbach & Rescorla, 2001) confirmed that Kayla was more angry and aggressive than most children her age, and had more difficulty regulating affect and controlling impulses. Given Mrs. B's overreporting of negative behaviors and general attitude of anger at Kayla, these results were given less weight than the school report. Kayla's second-grade teacher, who completed the teacher report version of the CBCL, was more positive about Kayla. She was noted to have strengths in the areas of leadership with peers, confidence, and academic aptitude. However, this teacher also noted general dysregulation and poor impulse control during unstructured periods of the day, in which Kayla's behavior had become increasingly disruptive.

Standardized Assessment of Sexual Behaviors

The CSBI (Friedrich, 1997) was incorporated into Kayla's assessment. As described throughout this book, the CSBI is an empirically supported measure utilized to obtain a caregiver's report of a wide range of sexual behavior in a child ages 2–12 years. The CSBI is based on the finding that sexual abuse is frequently related to the presence of precocious sexual behavior in children. This 38-item measure covers a variety of domains, including boundary problems, exhibitionism, gender role behavior, self-stimulation, sexual anxiety, sexual interest, sexual intrusiveness, sexual knowledge, and voyeuristic behavior (Friedrich, 1997). Exposure to nudity and sex were related to the CSBI total score in both the normative and clinical groups. (See Chapter One for a fuller discussion.)

Kayla's total CSBI score was elevated (T score > 110), as compared to those of similar-age female children. The CSBI total score is based on the subtotal scores in two domains. The first, Developmentally Related Sexual Behavior, reflects the child's level of age- and gender-appropriate behavior. Kayla's overall score on this scale was elevated (T score = 80). The second scale, Sexual Abuse Specific Items, contains items that are empirically related to sexual abuse history; these differ for boys and girls (Friedrich, 1997). According to Mr. and Mrs. B's report, Kayla scored significantly higher than her similar-age peers on this scale (T score > 110; at-risk range).

Initial Assessment Impressions

Kayla arrived for each weekly assessment session on time, accompanied by her mother and stepfather. The parents brought both of the younger children, and Mrs. B frequently appeared frustrated and overwhelmed in the waiting room—often yelling at her younger children or chasing after them when they wandered off down the hallway. Mr. B was observed to attempt quietly and passively to quiet the younger children and reassure Mrs. B, maintaining a calm and kind presence. (This often irritated Mrs. B.)

Kayla developed a rapport with me (J.A.S.) quickly, and her affect shifted significantly when she separated from her family. She often seemed frustrated or angry upon arrival and needed a few minutes to make the transition into the assessment hour. As part of this transition, Kayla engaged in 3- to 5-minute relaxation exercises, and I used a meditation chime to start and end our time together. Initially resistant, Kayla quickly embraced the relaxation period (both before and after the assessment session) and began asking to ring the chime to start the exercises (which included controlled breathing, progressive muscle relaxation, and guided visualization with a children's meditation CD).

In the first assessment session, Kayla was told why she was here and what I had been told about the behaviors at school that caused some problems. I told her that this was a place that helped children shrink "big feelings," which included feeling like touching private parts, or "touching feelings." I also told her that there were lots of kids who had touching feelings that turned into "touching problems," and that there were things we could do (in therapy) to make the feeling and the problem behavior smaller. Kayla was very attentive as I introduced her to the play environment, reviewed what we would do together, and noted why she had come to treatment. Kayla seemed surprised to hear that there were "lots of kids" with similar problems. I told Kayla that my first job was for us to get to know each other a little, and that my second job was to learn more about and then help her with the touching problem, which seemed to be causing problems for her at school and home. I also told her that I would like to understand where the touching idea came from and what usually made it grow bigger, to the point that it moved from a thought to a behavior. Kayla was very attentive to what I said, and then asked questions about other kids and "where their touching problems came from." Her interest and willingness to talk with me were noted as a little out of the ordinary. Other children take longer to warm up and often remain reserved for a number of sessions.

At the start of the second session, following a controlled breathing exercise and affective scaling check-in (rating and illustrating how she was feeling "right now"), Kayla had clearly thought more about the previous session: She had more questions about other kids' problems and very specific questions about private parts. Kayla was curious and seemed eager to pursue her curiosities in a safe, supportive environment. Most notable by this second session was how calm and focused Kayla was during discussions. It was in this session that Kayla disclosed several incidents with a 12-year-old male cousin (Tyler) in the summer prior to first grade. Kayla had spent several weeks with her maternal grandmother and cousin as part of a summer vacation. She had been 6 years old at the time, and Tyler was 6 years her senior. Kayla disclosed in a straightforward manner, "My cousin has a touching problem too, and he touched me *a lot*!" (giggling nervously). I responded that this could help explain why her touching feelings got so big so fast and became a problem. The rest of the second session and the third session were focused on these disclosures, including informing the parents; contacting child protective services; and conducting a therapy session with Kayla, her mother, and her stepfather. This disclosure, and the positive response Kayla received from her mother (after the mother had shared with me her initial disbelief and worry that Kayla might be lying), created a significant shift in Kayla's overall mood and behavior at home.

Structured Assessment Tasks

Play Genogram

As noted in Chapter Four, a "genogram" is a visual depiction of family members and their relationships that allows a clinician to understand the composition of a child's family, individual traits, and the nature of family relationships from the child's perspective. Typically, a genogram not only includes information about family composition, but indicates whether family members are dead or alive, whether there are divorces or adoptions, and the birth order of children. Kayla first decided who would be included in her family, and wrote down the following members: her mom, her dad, her stepdad, her siblings (Kaleb and Katie), and her second-grade teacher.

Kayla was then given the following directive: "Choose a miniature that best shows your thoughts and feelings about each person in the family, including yourself." Kayla proceeded thoughtfully and slowly through this activity. She was focused and seemed invested in finding the best fit for each member. Kayla selected for her stepfather and father first, and her mother last. For her stepfather, Kayla chose two miniatures: a small, playful bear and a briefcase ("because he's nice and has to work a lot"). For her biological father, Kayla chose a large male figure holding a small child on his shoulders ("because he loves to be with me and misses me"). For her siblings, Kayla chose a small toy for each, and a miniature of a baby crying ("because they cry sooo much"). For her teacher, she chose a tall female holding a book and smiling ("she likes me and I like her"). For herself, Kayla chose three miniatures: (1) a small monster-like figure ("because sometimes I'm mean"); (2) a teenage girl figure in revealing clothing, talking on the phone ("that's me, talking to my boyfriend"); and (3) a child on a bike ("I love to ride my bike"). For her mother, Kayla chose a large, female monster figure (a woman with open mouth and sharp teeth, wearing a cape). The largest figure chosen was for her mother, and the smallest figures were her stepfather and younger siblings. The three miniatures she chose for herself were all facing away from her mother and stepfather, and the mother was carefully placed facing and moving toward Kayla. Kayla's figure of herself on a bike was positioned as going toward the figure she chose for her biological father.

This play genogram revealed many of Kayla's underlying concerns and seemed congruent with some of what she and her parents had already shared with me. It was interesting to note that she chose to include both fathers, although her stepfather had been her primary father figure since she was 3½ years old. Kayla apparently harbored feelings of abandonment by her birth father and unresolved feelings about the separation. When she chose a miniature to show her thoughts and feelings about him, she chose a miniature that included herself and her father together; as a matter of fact, the child was being carried by the parent, and thus her longing for him was crystal-clear. She depicted her stepfather well, as playful and absent much of the time, and her siblings as attention-demanding and annoying (not atypical of sibling responses). Her mother's figure—large, facing in her direction, and aggressive—seemed to capture Kayla's sense of receiving much negative and hostile attention from a frustrated, angry mother. At the same time, she had a monster quality that was also visible in one of Kayla's choices for herself: On some deep level, Kayla probably wanted to find a connection between herself and her mother, and maybe the quality they shared at the moment was their aggression toward others. It was important to note that the mother's position facing Kayla had elicited Kayla's turning away; I noted that this was something we could revisit in therapy.

Finally, a few other issues seemed important in this play genogram. First, Kayla included a positive relationship with her teacher, showing her receptivity to being liked by someone and her capacity to reciprocate those feelings. Second, her preoccupation with boys and a desire to be a teen talking to a boyfriend was an interesting depiction of her understanding that it was older children who had boyfriends, not 7-year-olds. I made a mental note to reintroduce her three miniatures of herself later on and to use them as a bridge to three very important issues about herself: her wanting to rush ahead into relationship with boys; her seeing the problem behavior as monster-like; and her being on a bike, which could denote her desire to move faster (her apparent high energy). This play genogram also informed some of the therapy issues that would need focus—namely, her two primary relationships and her current difficulties with each. Kayla seemed a wonderful candidate for play therapy; her symbolic language was rich and informative.

Drawing Tasks

FREE DRAWING

If children express an interest in drawing or painting, they can be encouraged to "draw a picture of anything that comes to mind," or "anything you'd like to draw or paint." Kayla chose to use crayons and drew a boy and girl holding hands. She added, "That's me and my new boyfriend." Kayla then shared a "secret": that she had a boyfriend at school who was 10 years old. She described kissing on the playground, but she was not sure that this boy knew they were "dating." Kayla talked excitedly about this child and shared details of the "love notes" she gave him at school. Kayla stated that she drew him pictures of "sex," and described sex as "when a boy puts his thing in here [putting her hand between her legs]." When asked how she had learned about sex, Kayla responded, "I've known a long, long time."

KINETIC FAMILY DRAWING

As noted in Chapter Four, the instruction to the child for K-F-D is "Draw a picture of you and your family doing something together— some type of action." Children may ask about the term "family"— specifically, which family they should draw. Clinicians encourage children to draw whichever family they wish to draw. After children complete the task, clinicians ask children to say as much or as little as they want.

Kayla drew all members of her current household, including herself, and added her biological father. She drew stick figures and illustrated each one very similarly (identified by adding the person's name above each head), but she used a different color for each (Kayla's color for herself was black). Kayla completed this task quickly and chose not to embellish the drawing. When asked what the family was doing, Kayla said, "Nothing . . . that's just us." Her father was drawn as the largest figure, off to the side and next to Kayla. There was no ground line, as if all members were floating. All facial expressions were the same (e.g., a straight line for the mouth).

SELF-PORTRAIT

After children have had opportunities to make free drawings, they are asked to draw a picture of themselves. This directive is simple and straightforward: "Draw a picture of you." Kayla refused to do the self-portrait in the third session. She completed the drawing in the following session (it was laid out as the first activity, prior to time for free play), but she did so quickly and immediately turned the page over, stating, "I'm a horrible drawer. This is ugly!" She chose a black crayon. The picture did not include a body—just a large head with dots for eyes (drawn very small and out of proportion), small nose, ears, and again a straight line for a mouth. She added a few long strands of hair, but was becoming increasingly agitated, so she did this quickly and with frustration; at the end of her drawing, she flipped it immediately over and proceeded angrily to the sand tray. Kayla made the transition to the sand activity fairly quickly, but the self-portrait task created distress and a significant shift in affect.

Color Your Feelings

As described in Chapter Four, the Color Your Feelings assessment technique is designed to inquire about children's perceptions of their emotions and the intensity of these emotions. Specifically, children are asked to make a list of feelings they have most of the time, and then they are asked to pick a color that best shows that feeling. As shown in Form 4.2, a column of little boxes is placed next to the list of emotions; children fill in the little boxes with their chosen colors to create a personalized color code. After children create their individualized color code, they are given outlines of gingerbread figures (also included in Form 4.2) and are asked to fill in the outlines using their color code, indicating how small or large those feelings are when they experience "the touching problem" (or a situation related to a child's presenting problem). After this task is completed, children are asked to say as much or as little as they would like about what they have completed.

Kayla identified four feelings she had "most of the time" as (in this order): happy, mad, angry, and sad. She used small dots of color on a gingerbread figure as follow: happy (chest), mad (head/face), angry (lower leg), and sad (arm). She completed the task quickly (see Figure 7.1).

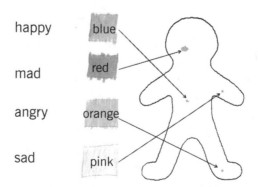

FIGURE 7.1. Kayla's feelings "most of the time."

Next Kayla was asked to illustrate the figure, again using her color code, for feelings she had "when you have the touching feeling." (I used the bus incident as an example: "like the feelings in your body when you touched him and told him to touch you.") Using the same colors for happy, mad, angry, and sad, Kayla used much more color and did so energetically.

When asked to illustrate the "touching feeling" and show where and how big it was in her body, Kayla placed her sad feeling at the top of her head (filling half the space); placed her happy feeling in her chest (the largest of the feelings depicted); placed her angry feeling on one arm, near her hand; and placed her mad feeling in between the legs (see Figure 7.2). Kayla chose not to say more about her picture.

During the treatment phase (supportive individual therapy before the start of a group for girls with sexual behavior problems), Kayla did another Color Your Feelings, using the same color code and following a similar directive. However, this time she was asked to show how where and how big or small her feelings were when she was hurt by her cousin's touching problem. As shown in Figure 7.3, her angry feeling replaced sad in the head region, and it filled the entire space of the figure's head. Her happy feeling was the largest depicted; it filled her chest, her torso, and parts of her arm. She stated that she was happy "because I hurt him . . . I pushed him off the bed." Anger was depicted again in between her legs. Sadness was small on this Color Your Feelings (a small dot of color on her hand). Kayla's primary feeling states when she thought about her own abuse were thus described in color as "mad" and "happy" (to have hurt her abuser too).

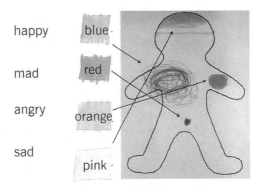

FIGURE 7.2. Kayla's feelings when she has the "touching feelings."

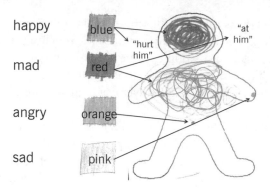

FIGURE 7.3. Kayla's feelings when touched/abused.

Sand Therapy

When sand therapy is used as an assessment task, a child is shown a rectangular box of specified dimensions, which is painted blue on the bottom and sides and is filled with fine, white sand. Near the box, there are a number of miniatures on shelves that are usually used in sand therapy. The child is shown the box and is told, "You may use as few or as many miniatures as you'd like to build a world in the sand." The child's spontaneous comments are documented, and the clinician remains a silent witness, assisting the child only when the child makes a direct request for assistance. After the child completes building a scenario in the sand, the clinician asks the child to say as much or as little as the child wants.

Kayla created two sand trays during the six assessment sessions we had, and the scenes were similar in both process and content. Kayla mostly enjoyed the sand tray work, and asked each session whether she would have time to work in the sand. By the sixth session, she was either asking to show the stories to and share them with her mom or requesting a picture of her completed project. Kayla interacted minimally while creating her worlds in the sand, and shared each story with full detail. The themes were dating scenarios: a girl and a boy on a date and the girl's process of getting ready for the date; and a girl and boy taking a walk for a date, kissing, and having "sex" at the end of the date. She took the most time setting up the "dates" and anticipating the boyfriend's arrival. No adults were present in her two sand scenarios. At the end of the second scenario (after putting the two miniatures on top of each other and making a kissing sound), Kayla added, "That's me and my boyfriend" (the 10-year-old boy she gave notes to at school). Her sexual preoccupation seemed to appear in almost every assessment task she undertook and became one of the treatment goals to address.

ASSESSMENT RESULTS

Kayla related comfortably to me and fully participated in the extended assessment process. She embraced mindfulness exercises at the beginning and end of each session, and could clearly convey negative perceptions of herself and of dysfunctional familial patterns through expressive arts (sand therapy, drawing tasks, the play genogram), nondirective play, and spontaneous comments. Kayla's disclosure of her own abuse and detailed reporting of her affective experiences when engaging in sexual behaviors provided her with near-immediate relief from the burden of carrying these experiences alone. As she began to play out and talk about her abuse, she demonstrated a shift in affect both in the sessions and at home. Mr. B told me enthusiastically that Kayla's overall mood was becoming steadier. Mrs. B was not yet able to notice or identify progress and minimized her husband's report by stating, "She never gives him a hard time; she saves her annoying self for me!"

Kayla's self-image had been deteriorating for several years prior to the escalation in sexual behaviors. Although she responded cooperatively to all the assessment tasks, she had the greatest reluctance to complete her self-portrait and approached this art task in anger, refusing to take her time or look at her finished product. As described above, she drew hurriedly; immediately flipped the picture, saying it was ugly; and literally walked away in near-disgust.

For nearly 2 years, Kayla's experiences of others had been those of abandonment, betrayal, and disregard of her emotional and interpersonal needs. Kayla's behavioral problems started escalating in the first grade, and these behaviors gradually isolated her from peers; gained negative attention from some teachers and her parents; and left Kayla with limited capacity to cope with overwhelming affect, confusion, and sexual feelings. She had struggled to resolve the wounds from her specific trauma (sexual abuse) on her own—without a secure base, without adult support in general, and without understanding or nurturance from her mother in particular. To add to her stressors, she felt abandoned by a biological father whom she idealized, and she held onto unrealistic ideas that he was longing for her as much as she pined for him. Her mother was overwhelmed by caring for two toddlers, and her energy seemed depleted. In addition, for whatever reasons, the mother seemed to view Kayla as unrewarding, demanding, and a constant source of tension in her life. These feelings had emerged shortly after Kayla was born; possibly Kayla was difficult to care for, or perhaps the mother was ambivalent about having a child at her young age, or with Kayla's father. The mother remained unwilling to speak too much of Kayla's father, so perhaps he was a source of pain to her in some way, and his daughter reminded her of this pain. Sometimes it's hard to understand how negative parental feelings emerge and persist, but it was clear that the mother found great dissatisfaction in her relationship with Kayla and that Kayla had begun to turn away from her mother, expecting little nurturing from her.

At the completion of Kayla's six-session assessment, the results revealed several serious issues that seemed to underlie, fuel, and maintain her current emotional difficulties, behavioral problems, and preoccupation with sexual topics. It was very clear that Kayla demonstrated excessive anger, dysregulation, and severe mood fluctuations. She also exhibited aggressive, intrusive, and oppositional behaviors at school and home. And her current sexual preoccupation resulted in her using sexualized and suggestive language, as well as aggressive sexual behaviors toward peers and younger children.

TREATMENT GOALS

The following treatment goals were set:

1. Address problematic attachment patterns in the mother–child relationship (developing since birth and exacerbated by untreated maternal depression, inadequate/inconsistent parenting, and the mother's overidentification of Kayla with negative attributes of her biological father).
2. Help the family cope with or resolve current family stressors (including the limited availability of the stepfather, whom Kayla viewed as her only nurturing caregiver; absent or unreliable emotional availability of the mother as the primary caregiver; and ongoing financial stressors).
3. Help Kayla address her unresolved abandonment issues related to her biological father's absence.

4. Assist Kayla to process the thoughts and feelings associated with her untreated sexual abuse.

It is important to underscore that Kayla was referred for services because another child's safety was compromised, not because of concern over her own consistent escalation in problem behaviors. This referral is typical of what we encounter in providing services to children with sexual behavior problems: The referring parties are concerned primarily with the safety of potential child victims, and not with what may be underlying the referred children's social, emotional, and behavioral difficulties. Unfortunately, steps such as punishing Kayla publicly, or suspending her from school, had only served to confirm her negative self-esteem. From Kayla's perspective, the immediate and intense response to a behavior that affected another child reinforced her perception that she was "bad" or "different," and hence less deserving of compassion and understanding. In response, Kayla's oppositional and aggressive behaviors worsened, and her mother's responses became increasingly inappropriate and emotionally abusive and neglectful.

TREATMENT PLAN AND PROCESS

Prior to treatment, Kayla's mother and stepfather participated in an assessment feedback session to discuss results and treatment recommendations. Mr. and Mrs. B were provided with formal oral and written reports; provided with general guidelines for parents of children with sexual behavior problems (see Form 5.1 in Chapter Five) and a supervision contract to be worked on at home and reviewed in the first family therapy session; an outline of recommended treatment goals as listed above; and a graphic describing the 12-session therapy program for sexual behavior problems in children (see Form 6.1 in Chapter Six).

Kayla and her family were assigned an ongoing social worker by the county department of family services, which had secured county funding for treatment of this family. The social worker had made a positive connection to Mrs. B, offering to help her in many ways that seemed useful to the mother—not the least of which was securing funds for therapy and babysitting services that the family could otherwise not afford.

The following recommendations were made to Mr. and Mrs. B, reflecting a comprehensive response to their daughter's behavioral problems, as well as their own stressors:

1. In-home counseling services to address Kayla's relationship to her mother and to begin to build positive interactions between them.
2. Parental counseling to cover safety and supervision issues, behavior problems, inappropriate parental response to behaviors, reinforcement of outpatient therapy goals, and at-home work on issues introduced in group sessions.
3. A 12-session commitment to once-weekly concurrent parent and child group therapy for children with sexual behavior problems, including a parent–child relationship enhancement component at the end of each session (the Boundary Project model; see Chapter Six).
4. Individual trauma-focused integrated play therapy for Kayla (Gil, 2012), following completion of sexual-behavior-specific treatment.
5. Attention to recommendations that would be submitted after parent and child therapists reported progress made during group therapy.
6. Increases in Kayla's prosocial after-school activities and opportunities for daily physical activity.
7. An immediate meeting of the therapist, case manager, and parents with Kayla's teacher, counselor, and principal—(a) to review current risk factors and current needs for increased support from school personnel; and (b) to provide psychoeducation as Kayla reentered the school environment in order to reduce risk to other children as well as the risk of Kayla's future expulsion.
8. Attention to child protective services' recommendations for no contact with Kayla's abusing cousin (Tyler) and for related legal action.
9. Individual weekly supportive therapy for the mother to include a psychiatric consultation to explore possible medication for mood disturbance.

As demonstrated by this treatment plan, a comprehensive response is necessary and appropriate in cases such as these, and it requires a team approach that no single professional can provide alone. Given the serious school and safety concerns about Kayla's increasingly aggressive sexual behaviors, the immediate goal was to provide Kayla with strategies to manage her sexual thoughts and feelings so that she would no longer be a risk to other children, including her classmates and siblings. To achieve this goal, Boundary Project objectives were introduced during group therapy, practiced during parent–child reviews at the end of each session, and reinforced at home between therapy sessions with specific activities designed to promote relationship building and improve emotional communication between Kayla and both her caregivers.

Unique aspects of our treatment approach include a focus on several factors usually not addressed in generic therapy, including provision of clear and consistent guidelines for creating a safe and appropriate environment. In Kayla's case, these guidelines included parental supervision of all Kayla's TV watching and other media consumption; coordination among school, home, and therapy; parental supervision of Kayla's interactions with her siblings; and increased monitoring of her play alone. In addition, we encouraged all care providers, across settings, to provide consistent and explicit messages to Kayla when they observed inappropriate behaviors. Given the amount of negative attention this child had received, and the fact that her self-esteem and identity had been gravely affected, we also encouraged all caretakers in all settings to respond to Kayla with kindness, so that she would feel valued, wanted, and (most of all) loved.

Several other strategies were to be implemented at home (relaxation and mindfulness strategies, affective identification and scaling, etc.). Kayla was happy to take the lead in asking her parents to do joint activities with her or eventually to show them plainly how she felt and how big or small her feelings were at any given time.

Mr. B, as usual, responded with optimism. Mrs. B took longer, given the other issues involved for her; however, as she participated in her own therapy and began to resolve some of the issues of her relationship with Kayla's biological father, her general demeanor began to change. The parent–child relationship seemed to show some changes for the better, but the pervasive distance between Kayla and her mother could not be overcome. Mrs. B did, however, begin to recognize Kayla's fighting spirit as an asset, and she eventually began to enjoy spending time with her. She also began to feel confident that Kayla could take care of the younger children, offering her welcome respites from time to time.

Therapy with Kayla went smoothly and progressed quickly. She was very responsive to clinical attention, and she remained cooperative and eager to participate throughout. We had a long-term therapy relationship that we both valued, and it took about 1½ years to achieve our goals; treatment was then terminated. During that time, Kayla discovered dance—and Mrs. B found a way to send her to weekly lessons, which endeared her mother to Kayla. She also found school a safe and warm environment once her problem behaviors were no longer causing a stir, and she settled into a more positive experience academically and socially. Probably the most pivotal experiences occurred when Kayla developed a friendship with another girl her age, and the two found in each other a source of warmth that grew in leaps and bounds—so much so that Kayla insisted in bringing Olivia to our sessions a few times. She wanted us to meet, since "you both like me and I like us both."

SUMMARY AND CONCLUSIONS

Kayla was a child not unlike many children who are referred to our clinic for specialized services in sexual behavior problems. The initial focus on these problems is usually balanced out by more information gleaned through the extended, developmentally inviting ASBPC process. In our experience, children are often surprised by our willingness to get to know them, listen to them, and provide understanding. Too often, children with sexual behavior problems are referred after their behaviors have become seriously problematic to others and those behaviors have elicited severe negative consequences, such as isolation, public punishments, or suspensions or expulsions. Parents have often dealt with guilt and shame, as well as confusion, despair, and fear about what is causing these behaviors to surface.

And just as in the example of Kayla, our assessments uncover a host of problem areas that need to be addressed, negating the idea that only the child needs to be "fixed"! Usually a child's behavioral problems stem from a host of unresolved issues—including difficult personal experiences; an overstimulating environment, including access to electronic and/or print media that provide explicit information beyond the child's ability to process; and family dynamics that either contribute to or maintain the problem in some way. Children with sexual behavior problems often feel a range of emotions that seem to overwhelm them. In Kayla's case, these included a sense of abandonment by and longing for her father, as well as confusion about her mother's negativity toward her. Family stressors included her stepfather's working too much away from home, her mother's desperation to make ends meet, and younger siblings who were demanding of parental attention.

Children with sexual behavior problems have not always been abused, but it seems that these behaviors are often associated with histories of abuse and/or with environments providing easy access to explicit sexual information that exceeds children's developmental abilities to integrate. In addition, inappropriate friendships can introduce inappropriate sexualized behaviors, as can witnessing sexual activity by older siblings or parents.

Finally, a host of interrelated factors must be considered in assessing and treating children with sexual behavior problems, and it is essential to provide comprehensive, collaborative, and meaningful responses to these factors. Treatment outcomes are greatly enhanced by obtaining primary caregivers' participation and investment, because without these adults' willingness to work to understand their children and respond in kind and appropriate ways, treatment will be stymied. Unless parents/caregivers make a substantial investment in their children's treatment (including attendance in parent groups and follow-up at home), either progress is impaired, or the reduction in sexual behavior problems is simply temporary, or the sexual behaviors are replaced by other negative behaviors or emotional problems.

The research supports our clinical experience that children with sexual behavior problems can be helped to stop their inappropriate behaviors; can learn to express themselves more fully and appropriately; and usually show great resiliency and trust, in spite of their pains, losses, and frustrations. Thus this work can be undertaken with enthusiasm and optimism.

CHAPTER EIGHT

The Case of Thomas

REFERRAL INFORMATION

Thomas M was a 4-year-old European American boy who was referred for a sexual behavior assessment by the director of his preschool. Within the past 2 months, Thomas had been sent home due to inappropriate touching of another child. Of primary concern to the school was Thomas's unresponsiveness to appropriate redirection when he attempted to kiss and hug classmates and teachers, to touch his penis and show it to classmates, and to lift the dresses of girls in the class. Although these behaviors were initially viewed as developmentally appropriate curiosity about body parts, the school staff was now concerned that there might be more serious issues at play for Thomas. The school director asked for an assessment that could explore sexual abuse as a possible cause of Thomas's sexualized play and inappropriate behaviors. According to his teacher, Thomas was starting to try to isolate other children and "hide what he's doing." Rather than being successfully redirected to another activity, Thomas seemed to be responding by pursuing his interest and curiosity in more private, secretive ways.

Thomas's preschool classmates had begun teasing Thomas and refusing to play with him because of these behaviors. School personnel also noted that he had begun responding more aggressively when classmates set limits and refused to play with him. At other times, Thomas withdrew, became disruptive, stood up and walked around, and seemed unwilling or unable to participate with the class. His teacher stated that Thomas "just leaves the situation defeated, shuts down for hours, and refuses to talk or play with the other kids. . . . He goes from hyper to shut down in a matter of seconds, and it takes a long time to get him back."

During a recent school meeting, Thomas's teacher proposed that the school obtain the services of a one-on-one assistant for him within the classroom, to ensure the safety of other children. In addition, his teacher suggested that Thomas be referred to an alternative school for his kindergarten year. Even though Thomas was considered cognitively advanced for his age, and had a history of success with classroom expectations, the school was not comfortable with promoting Thomas to kindergarten. Before the onset of his frequent sexual behaviors, Thomas had required assistance from the school for other difficulties, including dysregulation that inhibited his ability to pay attention or participate in classroom activities without one-on-one assistance from a teacher. Issues with physical boundaries also predated the sexual behaviors (e.g., shoving children while remaining seemingly unaware of their feelings, getting too close to peers and teachers, and on one occasion kicking a teacher when she attempted to redirect him).

At this time, Thomas resided in a therapeutic foster home—his second foster home in 13 months. He had been with his current foster family for approximately 6 months. The first had been a temporary placement until a therapeutic foster home could be found. Unfortunately for Thomas, he had grown attached to his first foster family (mother, father, and two teenage foster siblings), to the point that he asked to be adopted by them. One month after this request to his social worker, another placement was found, and without explanation he was moved to this other home. His transition to this new foster placement had been difficult, and he often mentioned wanting to return to the other family.

A clinical interview with Thomas's social worker and current foster mother revealed that approximately 2 months earlier, Thomas was discovered attempting to undress his 5-year-old foster sister, Nataly. Nataly later told her mother that Thomas had attempted to take her underpants down twice before, and that she did not want to get him in trouble because she was afraid he would have to leave the foster home. The foster mother noted that most of the time, Thomas and Nataly played well with one another, and the mother asserted that she had increased her supervision around the house and did not let them play together alone. She also told us that when she discovered Thomas undressing Nataly, Thomas initially appeared frightened and embarrassed; he then ran away, hid behind some furniture, and refused to come out for 2 hours. Subsequent questions about the incident by his foster parents and social worker yielded no additional information or disclosures, but Thomas's behavior changed: He became less verbal and increasingly defensive, angry, and aggressive. His foster mother stated matter-of-factly, "It's like he has no empathy or remorse, so I have to watch him all the time."

In addition, Thomas's foster mother expressed concern that Thomas seemed preoccupied with her breasts and buttocks, and that she repeatedly had to put him in time out for inappropriate touching. She further noted that Thomas had showed his penis in public, just as he did at school, and that he laughed nervously when his foster mother got angry at this. She added, "I have no idea how to get through to him. It's like he doesn't care and does it just to get me mad." The social worker suggested that Thomas's increased behavioral problems might be related to resuming visitation with his birth mother, and the foster mother concurred that Thomas seemed excited and "wound up" after visits with his birth mother.

PSYCHOSOCIAL BACKGROUND

A little over a year ago, at the age of 3½ years, Thomas had been removed from his biological mother's care after child protective services discovered that Thomas had been physically abused by the mother's live-in boyfriend. Ms. M was also a victim of physical and verbal abuse by this boyfriend, and ostensibly Thomas witnessed this domestic violence. When Thomas was in his mother's care, neighbors had reported frequent fighting, yelling, and witnessing the boyfriend physically shake and slap Thomas in the community park. According to the primary social worker, Ms. M had complied with all recommended services, actively participated in her own therapy with a domestic violence specialist, secured employment, and immediately cut off contact with her boyfriend when she learned that Thomas had been a direct victim of her boyfriend's abuse. At the time that child protective services referred Thomas for assessment, he had begun making the transition back to his mother's care, including overnight visits on weekends. He was scheduled to return home within 3 months.

Thomas was the only child born to his mother, who was 22 years old at his birth. Ms. M had been married for 1 year before separating from what she described as an abusive relationship with Thomas's father. According to Ms. M, Thomas's father was addicted to drugs and alcohol and was unable to provide for himself or his young family. Ms.

M took Thomas and left her husband after he physically assaulted her while using drugs in the home. Ms. M received housing and supportive services in a local shelter from the time Thomas was 9 months old until he was nearly 2 years of age. Ms. M then secured housing for herself and Thomas and started gaining stability in their lives before meeting her most recent boyfriend.

Thomas was reportedly born on time, with no prenatal or perinatal complications. However, his records included a statement by his mother that there was possible trauma during pregnancy, "when I [Ms. M] got pushed to the ground and kicked in the stomach when I was 5 months pregnant." She went to an emergency care facility, and luckily her examination did not reveal signs of acute trauma to the mother or baby. Prenatal care was limited, and medical reports indicated mild developmental delays in speech and language. Ms. M also reported that Thomas had always had difficulty falling and staying asleep (he did not sleep through the night until 13 months of age), had a poor appetite, and cried more than most infants she knew. Thomas had not achieved daytime control of his bladder until 6 months before the current assessment, at nearly 4 years of age, and enuresis was a near-nightly occurrence. Physically, Thomas was a healthy child, with no concerns about his fine or gross motor skill development; he had experienced no known major illnesses or accidents. Socially, he had been observed "playing too rough" with friends, although he sought out playmates and showed interest in other children. His peer relationships however, often reflected a lack of social skills, poor impulse control, and general inattention or lack of awareness of other children's physical boundaries. School reports suggested an impression that Thomas might meet the criteria for Asperger's disorder because of his social difficulties, but no specific signs or symptoms were listed. Cognitively, Thomas was reported to be performing above average in all areas of his current preschool curriculum. He mastered concepts quickly and was already reading. Teachers stated that he loved to read and most enjoyed hands-on science projects, but that difficulties arose when Thomas was involved in groups (he became overwhelmed).

Thomas had no current relationship with his biological father. He had started asking about his father, and asking to live with him, when he was placed in foster care. Reportedly, reunification with his father was hoped for in the next year, as the father was expected to complete court-ordered substance abuse counseling classes and had started providing financial support to Ms. M. He had also maintained contact with social workers and had been consistently participating in all facets of his own recovery. Ms. M was open to reunification efforts, with the conditions that he remain in therapy and that the visitation be initially supervised.

Thomas was transported to his seven weekly assessment appointments by either his social worker or his foster mother. Thomas's birth mother, Ms. M, met with me (J. A. S.) for an intake and exit interview. She appeared motivated, concerned, and willing to meet all court requirements, including cooperating with this assessment and then following directives to help her child make the transition to her full-time care. Ms. M was working with her own therapist and provided consent for the team to consult her for treatment-planning purposes.

Before I met Thomas and attended a meeting with his foster mother and social worker, I also arranged to visit his school and observe Thomas's behavior during a structured and unstructured period, as well as while he made a transition from one activity to another. Within a span of 1½ hours, Thomas sought out negative attention from teachers five times, pushed two children during a structured activity when asked to share markers with the group, and cycled from excitement when cooperating with one peer to aggression when another child attempted to join the dyad. When he was teased, Thomas left the lunch table and found a quiet corner to read a book. He then ignored the teacher as she attempted to coax him back to his lunch. No sexualized behaviors were observed, but he twice wrapped his arms around his teacher's legs and would not let go until she forcibly removed his arms. Redirecting Thomas when he sought intimacy or touch seemed to trigger anger and frustration, so his attempts to seek proximity or comfort backfired, and he seemed lost or confused after these incidents. When I spoke with his primary teacher after my observation of Thomas, she noted that my observations were consistent with her daily struggles with Thomas. She added, however, that she really enjoyed Thomas when he was "having a good day." She stated that he was creative, very bright, loving, and playful, and could be a leader in the class "when he wants to be."

ASSESSMENT PROCESS

Upon Thomas's referral for specialized services to "rule out sexual abuse," an ASBPC was recommended (see Chapter Four). This extended, play-based assessment was completed with Thomas in seven sessions.

The first step in the assessment process is to do an intake with referring professionals and obtain general and specific information from both oral and written reports. During the structured intake, I obtained a developmental history; academic and social information from the preschool teacher and director; and results from the following assessment measures: the CSBI (Friedrich, 1997); the parent report version of the CBCL for children ages 1½–5 years (Achenbach & Rescorla, 2000); and the TSCYC (Briere, 2005). I also observed Thomas in his school setting (as described above) and during our seven meetings, which involved his participation in a number of directive and nondirective play and expressive art tasks.

Thomas completed all structured tasks associated with the assessment and fully engaged in free and cooperative play with me. Thomas often invited me to be involved with his "superhero" scenarios (as partners committed to eradicating bad guys), and could spend the whole session in a Spider-Man or a Batman mask and cape. I was invited to be his assistant, or sidekick, or "spotter" for bad guys. Thomas energetically and dramatically hunted "bad guys" around the room.

Alternatively, he also enjoyed quiet play and orchestrated grand battle scenes between "good guys" and "bad guys." Thomas was fully engaged in setting up specific strategies for both teams, and seemed to take pleasure in the victories of the good team over the bad team. The good guys always overwhelmed the monsters or opposing soldiers in a dramatic final scene that seemed to delight Thomas. Some battle scenes were particularly violent, but not atypical for an energetic boy of 4 years of age who had also been exposed to video games in his previous foster home with much older children. Thomas's life experiences to date had probably magnified his interest in creating fantasies in which bigger, stronger, and scarier people with superpowers allowed him to become invisible, strong, large, or fierce; able to fly away from danger; and capable of seeing threats of danger from great distances.

As guided by the ASBPC, each session included a period of time for a structured task (a drawing task, sand therapy, or the Color Your Feelings task). A period of time was also reserved for observing and assessing Thomas's child-centered, nondirective play in a standard play therapy environment.

Standardized Assessment of Nonsexual Behaviors

As reported by the school and Thomas's foster mother, Thomas had difficulty regulating his emotions; had low frustration tolerance; and was easily overstimulated by noise, transitions, and close physical proximity to others. He could become aggressive when overwhelmed and/or when he felt misunderstood. His teachers consistently reported that he exhibited intrusive physical behaviors and had difficulty taking redirection. However, Thomas could do very well when he was in a calm environment, participating in play tasks that he had chosen and enjoyed, or receiving one-on-one attention from a classmate or adult.

Given Thomas's history of early abuse, loss, and separation from his mother, his foster mother was asked to complete the TSCYC (Briere, 2005), a parent report measure of posttraumatic stress and related psychological symptomatology. This measure covers a variety of domains, including anxiety, depression, anger, posttraumatic stress, dissociation, overt dissociation, fantasy, sexual concerns, sexual preoccupation, and sexual distress (Briere, 2005). According to his foster mother's endorsements, Thomas's scores were elevated in the domain of posttraumatic stress. Like the corresponding scale of the TSCC (see Chapter Seven), the Posttraumatic Stress scale of the TSCYC reflects symptoms such as intrusive sensations, thoughts, memories of painful past events, nightmares, cognitive avoidance of memories and negative thoughts, and fear of others. Scores within the clinically significant range included anxiety, dissociation, sexual concerns, and anger. Results from the CBCL for ages 1½–5 (Achenbach & Rescorla, 2000), also completed by his foster mother, confirmed that Thomas was less able to manage his emotions and impulses than similar-age boys, and that he related less comfortably with other children. Most significant on this measure were scales measuring anger, aggression, inattention, and social development.

Standardized Assessment of Sexual Behaviors

The CSBI (Friedrich, 1997) was incorporated into the current assessment. (See Chapters One, Two, and Seven for descriptions of the CSBI.)

Thomas's total CSBI score was elevated (T score > 85), as compared to similar-age male children. As described in Chapter Seven, the total CSBI score is based on the subtotal scores of two domains. The first, Developmentally Related Sexual Behavior, reflects the child's level of age- and gender-appropriate behavior. Thomas's overall score on this scale was significantly elevated (T score > 99). The second, Sexual Abuse Specific Items, contains items that are empirically related to sexual abuse history, and that differ for boys and girls (Friedrich, 1997). According to his foster mother's endorsement of behaviors within the past few months, Thomas scored slightly higher than his similar-age peers on this scale (T score > 65; elevated). These results, of course, were not interpreted in isolation; however, the scores did seem consistent with others' impressions that Thomas's sexual behavior problems were less likely to stem from sexual abuse and more likely to result from a combination of other abusive experiences (including physical abuse and witnessing of domestic violence against his mother) with challenges he had experienced since infancy. In particular, Thomas's assessment considered the possible role of trauma *in utero* (his mother had been kicked in the stomach); formal testing would be needed to assess possible brain injury during fetal development, which might be contributing to Thomas's poor impulse control (including sexual behaviors and problems with physical boundaries), difficulty regulating his emotions, and aggressive behaviors.

Initial Assessment Impressions

Thomas was initially reluctant to participate fully in the structured tasks of this assessment. For two sessions, he explored the room and seemed distracted and overwhelmed by the toy selection. He particularly enjoyed the sand tray; the miniature soldiers, knights, and superheroes; the superhero costumes; and a wooden castle filled with two teams of knights. By the third session, Thomas had honed in on the castle and created an elaborate scene that stretched to all areas of the playroom (surrounding the castle "grounds"). Once the scene was completed, Thomas said, "Now you're on my team and we have to protect the castle." For the next two sessions, Thomas guided me through an elaborate and detailed challenge of protecting the inhabitants of the castle and destroying all possible intruders. Thomas gave himself a broad range of superpowers and offered a few to me; I eventually became a full partner in the adventure. Once he was engaged with me in this play, and a working relationship began building with each joint adventure, I was able to engage Thomas in more structured tasks. For the remainder of the assessment, Thomas chose to do a structured task first and leave the remaining time for free play.

No behavior problems were observed during his assessment, perhaps because the setting and structure were consistent and predictable, and because Thomas had an adult's full attention without interruptions or the need to divide this adult's attention with other children. He made transitions in and out of the assessment hour quickly and well, other than needing more reminders at the end to help clean up. Sessions began and ended with 2 minutes of a quiet relaxation or grounding exercise.

Thomas's affect, after the first few sessions, covered a full range. He was playful, creative, inquisitive, and eventually honest and forthcoming about his thoughts, feelings, and perceptions. Structured tasks were completed quickly, clearly in an effort to start free play with me. Some boundary issues were noted at the start of one of the sessions: Thomas jumped on my lap during the breathing exercise; he ran and hugged my legs before ending the session; and he frequently stopped his play and sought proximity to me for a few moments before resuming the play. I did not interpret these incidents of touching or seeking closeness as boundary violations, but rather as moments that Thomas needed some reassurance or grounding from someone he was coming to trust as an interested and supportive figure.

In the third session, when Thomas was becoming more available and engaged after two sessions of exploration and solitary play, I talked to him about why he was coming to see me (attempts to do so in the first session had elicited minimal interest from Thomas). I told Thomas about the school observations I had done; I added that I knew about his two foster homes, about scary things that had happened to him when he was little, and about the fact that he had just started to visit with his mom again. Thomas listened intently, as we had just completed reading a relaxation story and sitting quietly. His body was calm, and he was interested.

I also shared that I knew about "touching and showing feelings" that were getting big and getting him into trouble at school and with his foster mom. Thomas paused a few moments, then said, "Did they tell you about Nataly, too?" He seemed embarrassed, but was able to keep sharing and listening. I told Thomas that I had heard about his pulling down Nataly's pants, but I thought he and I could talk about these things when he kept coming to the office to see me. I told him that we would work on these problem behaviors together, including with his mother, so that she would know how to help him after he moved back home. He said, "So they go away forever? . . . OK," and then said, "Now it's my turn," as he hopped up and began constructing a castle scene.

Structured Assessment Tasks

Play Genogram

As described in Chapters Four and Seven, a genogram allows a clinician to understand the composition of a child's family, individual members' traits, and the nature of family relationships from the child's perspective.

Thomas chose to include many extended family members, current teachers, and pets from his two foster homes. He was then asked to help make a place for each person, using a circle for each girl, a square for each boy (including himself), and a square with a triangle on top for each pet. Thomas wanted to do this by himself, and seemed to enjoy mastering the directions and correctly creating circles for girls and squares for boys to show the people in each family.

Once the basic genogram was completed, Thomas was asked to "choose at least one miniature for each person that best shows your thoughts and feelings about that person." Thomas stayed on task for the very detailed project, which was made longer than usual by the number of family members he included in his play genogram. He persisted and made at least one miniature selection for each person. Thomas started to struggle when he looked for a miniature for himself: He became active and agitated, moved quickly about the room, grabbed groups of miniatures from shelves, and dumped them onto a square he identified as his own. All other family members had one or a few miniatures, carefully selected and intentionally positioned, but Thomas was unable to narrow down his choices for himself and became dysregulated. (See Figure 8.1.)

Following the activity, I used the chime to signal a transition to a calm, quieting activity. Thomas needed a few minutes to settle down, and I waited with him before he sat next to me and shared his thoughts and feelings about his play genogram. He did not say much about his selections other than giving fairly literal reasons for some of them, which is typical with children this young. I then commented, "Thomas, you seem to have a lot—a lot of miniatures on your square, more than anybody else." He said quietly, "I couldn't find something for me. I have lots of different parts of me." I told him he had shown lots of parts in a really good way by using lots of miniatures. He seemed to like this acceptance of his struggle to find just one. Finally, I offered, "Sometimes when we're trying hard and can't do it just the way we want, we can get lots of big feelings inside that grow." When I asked him to pick the feeling that he had felt trying to find a miniature to show him, he pointed to "angry" and said that this angry feeling was at the highest level of intensity, a 5 (see Form 5.2, the Affective Scaling Worksheet). Thomas and I agreed that we were going to work on keeping his difficult feelings at lower numbers and trying to make his positive feelings stay at high numbers. This session ended with a mindfulness exercise (deep breathing combined with a relaxation story for young children), and Thomas cozied up to me on the couch.

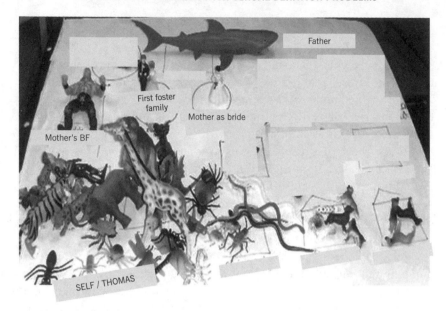

FIGURE 8.1. Thomas's play genogram: "I have different parts of me."

Drawing Tasks

FREE DRAWING

In the free-drawing task (see Chapters Four and Seven), Thomas chose to use a black marker and drew a series of shapes. He became frustrated a few times; he eventually went and selected a Spider-Man miniature and attempted to copy the design of the mask. He did not add color, but paid particular attention to the web design within the mask. When he finished, he simply handed the picture to me and said, "It's Spider-Man." He seemed pleased with his efforts and asked to take it home at the end of the session.

KINETIC FAMILY DRAWING

In K-F-D (see Chapters Four and Seven), the child is directed to "Draw a picture of you and your family doing something together—some type of action." In cases like Thomas's, the clinician encourages the child to draw whichever family member the child wishes to draw. After the child completes the task, the clinician asks the child to comment freely.

Thomas drew shapes of the following family members: himself as very small and between two figures he later named "Mom" and "Dad." Thomas used a red crayon for all family members. The style and proportions were consistent with the drawings of young children. However, no figure was complete with either arms or feet; dots were used for the eyes and noses of all three figures; and no mouth or facial expression was indicated on any figure. This lack of detail could have occurred because Thomas completed his art in a hurried, straightforward manner and immediately asked for his time to play. When asked what the family members were doing, Thomas said, "They are home, watching TV."

SELF-PORTRAIT

After children have had opportunities to make free drawings, they are asked simply, "Draw a picture of you." Thomas approached this task in much the same way as he approached other drawing tasks—quickly, with intention, and ready to move on to free play. Thomas returned to the box of pretend play clothes and masks and selected a Power Ranger mask. Thomas then again used shapes and fine lines (in black, thin marker) to draw the mask. He started over twice, but did not give up. He finished his project and said, "I'm a Power Ranger!"

Color Your Feelings

The Color Your Feelings assessment technique is designed to inquire about children's perceptions of their emotions and the intensity of these emotions. Specifically, children are asked to make a list of feelings they have most of the time, and then they are asked to pick a color that best shows that feeling (see Chapters Four and Seven, as well as Form 4.2).

With assistance from a picture book with a list of feeling names and feeling faces, Thomas identified five feelings he had most of the time, in the following order: sad, excited, angry, happy, and worried. Thomas then selected a color for each feeling and seemed interested in this task. When asked to show how small or big these feelings were in his body, Thomas seemed to understand the directive and started shading the gingerbread figure without questions or comments. He worked thoughtfully and quietly, using crayons, and took more time with this task than with the three drawing tasks described above. For feelings "most of the time," Thomas placed excited feelings in his hands and crown of his head; sad feelings on the tips of his toes and knees; angry feelings in his throat;

happy feelings in his chest; and worried feelings everywhere that white space remained. Once this art task was complete, Thomas commented that his worry was "biggest" because he was worried about his mom. His anger was the next largest feeling in his body, "because people are mean to me and I get *so* mad I want to scream in my mouth." He added that he was happy in his chest because "that's where my heart is and my mom loves me there."

Thomas completed a second Color Your Feelings in the following session. Using the same affective color code, Thomas was asked to show how his feelings might change from "most of the time" to when he felt his "showing problem" (which I described to him as the times when he took his penis out of his pants and tried to show it to his foster mom or classmates). Thomas again worked intently and seemed to grasp the directive. The difference was striking! This time, Thomas's primary (largest) feeling was excitement, and he shaded this in the torso, in the upper legs, and between the legs of the gingerbread figure. He added happy feelings to his hands; worried feelings to the top of his head ("because I might get in trouble"); and angry feelings again in his throat. Thomas did not add sadness to this Color Your Feelings, stating, "I'm not sad when I do that."

Thomas was able to talk a few minutes about his "showing and touching problem" immediately after this exercise. He was clearly able to identify shifts in affect and seemed to understand emotional intensity and how this can change when people think and do different things. Thomas approached this task with much more sophistication and apparent insight than most 4-year-old children do. Given this experience with Thomas, I continued to build on his affective color code (i.e., I expanded the range of emotions and corresponding colors), and I used Color Your Feelings regularly to check in with Thomas as he navigated transitions.

Sand Therapy

Thomas approached the sand therapy assessment task (see Chapters Four and Seven for general descriptions) similarly to his castle play: He first gathered all available knights from the miniature shelf, and then divided them into two teams. He then played out a battle scene, with the same themes he used in his free play (competition, good guys vs. bad guys, the inclusion of superpowers to help the good guys, and looming threat and protection from the bad guys). He then played out his story in the sand, describing it along the way. In the completed scenario, the bad guys were lying down as a group on one side and the good guys were standing erect. Once the play war was over, Thomas proceeded to bury the fallen knights, stating, "Now they are gone forever." Thomas immediately moved from the sand therapy task to free play involving superheroes, and he donned a cape and Captain America mask. Thomas's approach, process, content, and thematic material in this task were typical for boys his age.

ASSESSMENT RESULTS

Thomas settled into the play environment, where he was provided permission, space, and time to become comfortable with the setting, with the materials, and with me as the therapist. His initial reservation and solitary play in the first few sessions were replaced with shared interactions and mutual play that he guided. He had no difficulty making transitions away from his foster mother or social worker, and each informed me that he was excited to come to appointments after the second session, but he refused to answer their questions about what he did in his sessions.

I provided a structure for our time together that Thomas liked: He would choose an activity for half the session, and I would direct the other half. Thomas came to trust that each session would allow him to do some of what he wanted after or before the directive session, which dealt with one of his feeling or touching problems. Initially, Thomas complied with the structured beginning and ending routines (affective scaling and brief mindfulness exercises). By the third session, Thomas was initiating the use of the meditation chime to signal transitions, and he started to choose the book we would read. By the fifth session, Thomas wanted to be the reader and appeared pleased to show me that he was able to read (he smiled proudly at the end).

Difficulties in recognizing physical boundaries were apparent during the mindfulness exercises, when we sat closely together. Thomas sought physical touch and affection, but often a brief touch or reassuring response in return (pat on the back, holding his hand, or talking to him with a hand on his shoulder) resulted in his becoming more relaxed and attentive. Throughout, I took opportunities to connect types of touch to feeling words in preparation for treatment, which would explore his "touching problem" and his history of physical abuse. At the same time, I tried to set the context that some types of touching were appropriate.

Thomas's foster mother seemed to approach Thomas rigidly, and this was apparent in the waiting area. She seemed to focus on negative behaviors and seemed to anticipate a behavior problem as soon as Thomas emerged from his session (e.g., "Now remember we don't play when you finish; we leave and walk quietly to the elevator"). Once I noticed that she gave Thomas a long, firm lecture about his hand resting on her knee when they were reading a story in the waiting area before a session. When his foster mother lectured him, Thomas pulled away, folded his arms, and refused to look at the book. The foster mother continued talking to him about asking permission before touching a grownup. From Thomas's perspective, it must have seemed that the foster mother saw all touch as potentially problematic, since his attempts to seek security and affection were immediately redirected. Indeed, it appeared that all caregivers and teachers were focused on Thomas's not touching anyone unless they initiated the touch or he asked in advance. All of the caregivers meant well, and their intent was to help Thomas recognize physical boundaries. However, their focused and exaggerated responses were confusing to Thomas, who often seemed only to be seeking out human affection and emotional connection.

Thomas was a child who had experienced multiple losses, transitions, and traumas before the age of 4 years. He was a victim of physical abuse, including *in utero* violence by his father. After his mother was able to separate herself from his father, her boyfriend also exhibited violent behaviors, witnessed by Thomas between the ages of 2 and 3½. His only source of consistent security and comfort was his mother; it appeared that their relationship was close, and that she was affectionate and patient with Thomas, although she seemed passive and meek because of her own traumas. Child protective services removed Thomas from his mother's care because of the domestic violence with her boyfriend and her failure to protect Thomas. The abrupt removal from his home and mother left Thomas confused and attempting to navigate all these changes without his secure base and with uncertainty about when he would be allowed to visit or live with his mother. Thomas was placed in two foster homes, and he felt more comfortable in his first foster home. His subsequent placement with the current foster mother was stressful; his foster mother seemed rigid, rule-oriented, and negatively focused on Thomas's wrongdoing.

After his placement in the second foster home, Thomas became more aggressive. In particular, his sexual behaviors—especially showing his penis in public, or touching and peeking at classmates—provoked immediate and dramatic responses from his caretakers, who often removed Thomas from the situation, talked to him alone, and stayed in close proximity to him (including holding his hand when walking to and from activities). His identity in both his classroom and his foster home seemed to be limited to that of a child in need of supervision. Thomas's increasing aggression and escalation of sexual behaviors, including the recent sex play with his foster sister, suggested that Thomas was not able to make sense of these changes and was starting to see himself as potentially dangerous.

The assessment of his play suggested that Thomas was attempting to work out conflicting feelings. The battles he played out were dramatic, required the inclusion of superpowers, and included very large threats from multiple directions. As the key player in his stories, Thomas had to be vigilant, to control or "lead" his fellow knights or soldiers into safety, and to take control of the battles that ensued. Each story ended with the bad guys losing or the intruders being captured, caged, or buried in the sand.

After the assessment was complete, I held two feedback sessions: one with the social worker and foster mother and another with the birth mother, Ms. M. My primary recommendation to them all was to work on responding to Thomas's touching as his need to feel secure and valued. The risks of not responding to Thomas's requests appropriately were reviewed, despite some protest from the foster mother, who continued to assert that "Thomas is one of those children who needs lots of structure and clear rules of behavior."

I shared with them some of the research regarding the effect of witnessing domestic violence and physical abuse on young children, including what we now know about the relationship between domestic violence and sexual behavior problems. I reassured everyone that there was no indication of Thomas's being sexually abused, and that if this did turn out to be a factor, it would likely emerge in play therapy treatment sessions. Thomas's mother (Ms. M) responded with appropriate concern and immediately asked questions about what she could do specifically to help him. She seemed relieved to hear that Thomas needed her physical touch and expressions of affection more than ever, not less, because of his sexual behavior problems. We talked about ways to reinforce healthy touches and help Thomas recognize when his touches were inappropriate with herself or others. Given her response and willingness to help, and the fact that his return to her care was already in progress with overnight visits, I recommended that Ms. M be directly involved with Thomas's treatment. She assured me that she would attend every session and would cooperate fully with his treatment. She seemed grateful for the opportunity to participate, and seemed eager to obtain more information about Thomas and ways she could help him navigate these issues.

TREATMENT GOALS

The following treatment goals were set:

1. Provide psychoeducation to the current foster mother by conducting two parent sessions with her and Ms. M (with the social worker present). Psychoeducation would include information on children's emotional needs, sexual behavior problems in young children, and available research regarding prognosis and appropriate interventions.
2. Address Thomas's sexual behavior problems in individual therapy by taking an integrative approach, to include expressive arts and CBT.
3. Conduct individual sessions with a parent component to address sexual behavior problems within a family context. These sessions would include time for relationship-building exercises and would end with activities promoting healthy touch (e.g., Theraplay activities; Booth & Jernberg, 2010).
4. Request school personnel to collaborate with treatment and provide treatment-based interventions in the school setting (e.g., a "calming box" in his classroom to offer Thomas time, space, and materials/tools to self-soothe, regroup, and express his emotions to his teacher and other in-school caregivers).
5. Complete a neurological evaluation to rule out head trauma, given the history of physical abuse *in utero* and some symptoms that could be consistent with possible brain injury (poor impulse control, mood instability, aggression, inattention).
6. Conduct child-centered, nondirective play therapy following specialized treatment for sexual behavior problems. This treatment would assist Thomas to resolve his own traumas, including the early loss of his biological mother and father, as well as related issues upon reunification with his mother (and possibly his father).

TREATMENT PROCESS

Thomas and his mother participated in a 12-week course of specialized treatment for sexual behavior problems in young children (the Boundary Project). As described in Chapter Six, this treatment included focused attention on affect identification and expression; identification of appropriate and inappropriate touches; tools and strategies to address poor impulse control; a review of the cognitive triangle using a playful cartoon to illustrate problem illustrations and solutions (Thinkafeeladoo; see Figure 8.2); and parent–child relationship enhancement activities (Booth & Jernberg, 2010).

Thomas was not considered a candidate for group therapy at the time of this assessment. The reports of his caregivers, as well as my observation, indicated that Thomas found large groups overstimulating and that he did not have the skills to appropriately manage multiple demands on his attention or to share his therapist with other children. Once Thomas developed more tools and strategies to enable him to navigate social situations, a social skills group might be beneficial.

Boundary Project interventions can be delivered in either an individual, a group, or a family format (as described in Chapter Six), and parents or other primary caregivers are required to participate in all formats. Ms. M attended each weekly session and remained eager to follow recommendations. She and Thomas reported full use of the at-home reinforcement exercises, and she reported feeling more confident in her parenting. Ms. M was provided with a packet of psychoeducational materials and embraced all of these materials, including literature regarding attachment, child development, and brain-based parenting approaches. Thomas seemed thrilled to have his mother join him in his sessions; he still guarded his nondirective playtime, so extra time was provided at the end of each session for Thomas to choose a play activity with his mother. Thomas invited his mother into his play each time, and she became his trusted ally in the storytelling and superhero adventures.

SUMMARY AND CONCLUSIONS

Thomas was a 4-year-old boy who had survived multiple adverse situations, including witnessing domestic violence by two adult males, removal from his home by child protective services, two foster placements, and a great deal of negative attention as a result of his emotional

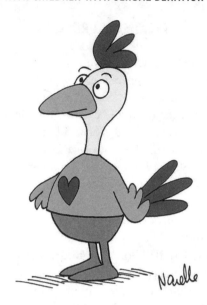

FIGURE 8.2. Thinkafeeladoo. Reprinted with permission from Brian Narelle.

and behavioral dysregulation. Thomas had demonstrated a host of behavioral problems, including physical aggression and sexual acting out. In particular, Thomas seemed to overlook physical boundaries and often exhibited intrusive behaviors toward peers and caretakers alike.

Staff members at Thomas's school had been patient and sought assistance in managing Thomas's behavioral problems. However, their patience wore thin as Thomas's problems increased, and as his sexual aggression took center stage and elicited grave concern. Although his second foster home seemed adequate and safe, his foster mother appeared to have low expectations and increasing distrust of Thomas. Thus both his school and home settings focused on his behavioral difficulties and left his underlying emotional needs unattended.

Thomas's primary attachment figure was his birth mother, Ms. M, who had been in two abusive relationships. To her credit, she extricated herself from both relationships, but not quickly enough to prevent Thomas's exposure to family violence. At the time of the referral, Thomas was renewing visits with Ms. M and expected to be reunited with her soon.

In both the assessment process and his later treatment, Thomas responded well to individual attention, and his reluctance to talk about his problem behaviors seemed to decrease as he gained trust in a clinical setting. Providing Thomas with a predictable setting in which he would be allowed to play out his concerns, ask questions, and talk about himself to the extent that he was able or willing seemed to comfort him greatly.

Both Ms. M and Thomas eventually participated in individual therapy with a conjoint meeting at the end of each session. During this time, they both received education and tools to begin to manage Thomas's dysregulation.

This case highlights the fact that some children act out sexually not because they have experienced sexual abuse, but because they have been exposed to overstimulating, violent environments that cause them intense internal distress. In addition, for young children of Thomas's age, exposure to so many transitions and losses can leave them unequipped to understand or negotiate their thoughts and feelings.

Thomas needed his mother to anchor himself in a secure attachment and then to help him to navigate his emotional life, in which rejection, loss, and lack of positive attention and nurturing were uppermost stressors. The knowledge that he and his mother would soon reunite provided optimism for Thomas and made him more receptive to using alternative ways to convey his distress.

CHAPTER NINE

The Case of Jenna

REFERRAL INFORMATION

Jenna was a 7-year-old Hispanic girl who was referred to child protective services after her 5-year-old brother, Roberto, disclosed to his kindergarten teacher that he did not want to go to the bathroom because Jenna had stuck her finger in his anus and it hurt him. The school social worker contacted child protective services, concerned that Roberto appeared to have a physical injury; after a preliminary investigation in which the service agency discovered Jenna's age, she was referred to our clinic for a "psychosexual evaluation."

Psychosexual evaluations are standard fare for adolescents and adults who commit sexual offenses. These evaluations consist of face-to-face interviews, psychological testing, and in some cases the use of polygraphs (more controversial in legal proceedings and less so for clinical use in treatment settings). Clearly, it would be impossible to evaluate young children with these adolescent and adult procedures, which rely so much on self-report and verbal communication. Thus, when referrals are requests for psychosocial evaluations, we provide a rationale for using a developmentally appropriate way to understand children's sexual behavior problems, such as the ASBPC process explained in Chapter Four. As described there, the ASBPC typically relies more on primary caregivers' reports and collateral information from other caretakers than evaluations of adolescents or adults do. In addition, children are invited to develop a relationship of trust and comfort with trained clinicians, who then do an extended assessment utilizing a broad range of directive and nondirective strategies, as well as a systemic/contextual lens to view the problem and responses to date.

PSYCHOSOCIAL BACKGROUND

Jenna was living with her maternal aunt, Alicia, age 39; her 5-year-old brother, Roberto; Alicia's husband, James, 42; and their son Phillip, 17. Alicia was the older sister of Glenda, Jenna's mother. At the time of the referral, Glenda was 23. She had delivered Jenna when she was 16 and Roberto when she was 18.

Alicia and James were approaching middle age at the time of this referral and were reliable caregivers to Jenna and Roberto, who had been living with them consistently for nearly 3 years. Alicia specified that Glenda had had trouble with drugs since her teen years, had become pregnant by two different men (she knew Roberto's father from Glenda's high school, but Jenna's paternity was unknown), and had felt unable to deal with taking care of her children. Glenda herself had been in the foster care system, but she was removed after her mother filed a Person in Need of Supervision petition, had a brief foster home placement, and then was placed in a group home for youth with behavioral problems. She ran away from the group home after a period of time and either lived with friends or slept on the street or in shelters. After Glenda gave birth to Jenna, she moved in with Alicia and seemed to settle down for a few months, but shortly thereafter she began to wander around with the child, unable to find a place to live or get a job. Alicia and James were in a position to offer shelter, but they set some limits on Glenda in regard to her using drugs and bringing strangers to the house; they also asked her to focus on Jenna and provide consistent caregiving. Unfortunately, Glenda had limited parenting capacities and was not motivated to get into a drug treatment program, so her judgment about her infant child was doubly impaired. Unwilling to take chances with Jenna's safety, Alicia used a "tough love" approach. She often explained to Glenda the dangers of putting her child at risk and reminded her of her own history in foster care. Eventually Glenda's behavior deteriorated, and in moments of sobriety she became terrified of losing her child, so she chose to ask Alicia to take more and more care of Jenna until she (Glenda) could get on her feet. Unfortunately, while Jenna was an infant and toddler, Glenda was drifting in and out of the house in various states of drug intoxication and dishevelment. Alicia began to notice that Glenda's visits became difficult for Jenna, as she often cried when her mother disappeared or showed up suddenly.

Alicia was alarmed when Glenda became pregnant again, this time talking idealistically about a high school sweetheart and the possibility that they would marry and live together. Alicia later found out that this young man was already married, estranged from his wife, and father to an infant. He and Glenda had met through their common interest in doing drugs and staying up all night. Needless to say, their plans to become a family never worked out; when Roberto was born, this young man left the state and never recognized Roberto as his son. Glenda was devastated when he disappeared, and she spiraled into more drug use and homelessness. She asked Alicia to take Roberto—who was born prematurely, underweight, and with substances in his system, so he was kept in the hospital and placed in foster care for the first few months of his life. Alicia made herself known to social services personnel, and after they conducted a home study, they placed 6-month-old Roberto in her care. In doing the home study, they also found that Alicia was taking care of Jenna informally, and so they referred her to an attorney to become a legal guardian for both children.

Glenda called Alicia a few times to ask after the children, but never gave any indication that she was interested in becoming their full-time parent; she was clearly unable to take care of herself. Alicia gave her numerous referrals to rehab programs, which Glenda agreed to attend, but she never followed through. Neither Alicia nor the social worker had much luck getting Glenda to respond to court requirements and/ or requests for regular visitation with her children. When I (E. G.) first met Jenna, she saw Alicia and James as her parents and seemed angry at her "real mom," who didn't come to see her regularly. As a matter of fact, procedures were under way for termination of Glenda's parental rights, and Alicia and James were going to become Jenna and Roberto's adoptive parents. Alicia had two jobs, a working husband, a successful marriage, and a self-sufficient life. Alicia and James had wanted a large family, but complications after the birth of their son, Phillip, had kept them from having more children. They were very invested in their niece and nephew, and they were raising them in a strong faith-based environment, which provided Jenna and Roberto with structure and limits as well as support.

When I first met with Alicia to talk about Jenna's presenting problems as well as her strengths, she jumped at the chance to give her family narrative. It appeared that Alicia had never really had a chance to talk about her feelings about Glenda, the upcoming hearing for termination of parental rights, and her love of and investment in Jenna and Roberto. As I listened to Alicia's account of her life while growing up, as well as her perceptions of what had happened to Glenda, it became clear that Alicia was a strong and centered woman with a great deal of affection toward her sister, but also appropriate frustration, concern, and anger. At this time, she confided that her major concerns were Jenna, Roberto, and Phillip, and her interest in doing whatever it took for them to have a more stable life and a good start that might ensure a better future.

Alicia reported to me that Glenda had been in trouble "all her life," because of her early drug abuse and unwillingness to go to school and study. Alicia believed that Glenda was negatively affected by their parents' divorce and the fact that she had to live alone with their mother at a critical time in her early teens. At the same time that Glenda was starting to get into a lot of trouble, Alicia and Glenda's mother was working two jobs; when she was home, she was sleeping and unable to look after Glenda. Alicia stated firmly that "my upbringing was absolutely nothing like my sister's, and everything fell apart when my father left." She added, "I was lucky that he chose to take me with him, because I was older and I could help him around the house." Alicia went on to say that her father had a 9-to-5 job, was always home to help her with homework, and eventually remarried someone Alicia saw as a "great role model, an elementary school teacher, and someone who inspired me to go to college." Alicia stated that her father "gave up" on Glenda and stated firmly that "she will never be right until she stops her drug habit." He also had little contact with her because he felt that Glenda was in with "a bad crowd," and wanted Alicia away from her influence as well. Alicia described her mother as a "good woman, a great heart," but unable to set limits and unprepared to face a world alone. Later on she confided that her mother had always had a drinking problem, and that Alicia suspected she had a history of depression. She noted that her father always spoke about her mother's drinking problem as always well hidden, but pointed to her depression and lack of interest in anything in particular, which caused her to withdraw from him and her children as they got older.

As Alicia went on to describe Jenna's early life, it became clear that Jenna had been exposed to an inconsistent, erratic, and drug-addicted parent who put her drug use first. Glenda had lived with her child on the streets, and it was likely that Jenna had been neglected (she was once found by a woman passing by on the street, bundled up in a dirty blanket), had witnessed domestic violence and adult sexual activity, and had gone through periods of fending for herself. Alicia had done the very best she could to stabilize Jenna's environment after she took Jenna into her home, but Glenda often took her young daughter back for brief periods of time (2–3 weeks). Because Alicia did not have any legal standing with her niece at that time, she felt she could not prevent Glenda from taking her child, but she did make sure that Glenda was sober when she took her daughter. Once Roberto was born and Alicia was counseled to take legal guardianship of both children, Alicia was able to exert more authority about Jenna's seeing her mother, but there were still times when Glenda showed up, took Jenna on unscheduled visits, and did not return her when she said she would. Alicia was initially reluctant to contact authorities and would go out looking for Glenda and her child. Luckily, there were specific places where Glenda usually went, and Alicia became proficient at finding her quickly. Eventually a court order prohibited Glenda from having unsupervised visits with her children. Alicia had to supervise all visits, which she did gladly.

Alicia reported that Glenda had begun drinking heavily at 10 years of age, added almost daily marijuana use in her teens, and later began using harder drugs. She emphasized that Jenna went "off the hard stuff" when she knew she was pregnant, but when she wasn't pregnant, she would have periods of "crazy, wild behavior." "It's a wonder she didn't get killed by someone on the streets. When she was tired or passed out from drugs, she simply lay down and slept." Alicia also noted that the streets are not a kind place to live with children. Glenda had talked about being raped on the street once; her few possessions were often stolen; and although food was shared, sometimes it was dirty, and many people shared germs and illnesses. Alicia finished talking about this part of Jenna and Roberto's history by saying, "I thank God that Jenna was not kidnapped or assaulted by someone out in the street. God is great."

It was clear from the data-gathering meeting with Alicia that she was an invested parent; that she had done all she could to provide Jenna and Roberto with a stable home; and that their birth mother, Glenda, had struggled with drug addiction most of her life and had a history of unwillingness or inability to take care of herself, much less her children. It also appeared that Glenda had been somewhat careful about not using drugs during her first pregnancy with Jenna, but did not do the same with her second pregnancy. Roberto had been born with symptoms of drugs in his system and had gone through an intense withdrawal. Thus Alicia understood that Roberto was likely to have special needs because of his mother's drug use during pregnancy, and that Jenna was also likely to have some difficulties, given her early life experiences with a young mother incapable of taking care of herself and a baby. Glenda's strength had been her willingness to reach out for help from her sister, Alicia, as she began to realize that she was not able to protect her young children. Neither Jenna nor Roberto had any contact with their biological fathers; indeed, only one of the fathers was known.

ASSESSMENT PROCESS

Caregiver Interview and Standardized Assessment of Sexual Behaviors

In regard to the sexual acting out that had caused the school referral to child protective services, Alicia said that Jenna had always had some unusual behaviors—touching herself frequently, using dolls to mimic sexual intercourse, and using inappropriate sexual language that showed she had explicit knowledge of sexual activity unusual for her age. When Alicia filled out the CSBI (Friedrich, 1997), the Sexual Abuse Specific Items score for Jenna's behavior was in the clinical range, indicating that her sexual acting out was unusual for her age and gender. Specifically, Alicia had endorsed items that had to do with masturbatory behavior and documented that it had been present since Jenna was a toddler. Alicia imagined that this was due to her unknown early experiences, but also wondered what she had seen during the unscheduled visits that Alicia had allowed with Glenda until recently ("God only knows what Jenna has seen and lived through"). Alicia had handled the masturbatory behavior by slapping Jenna's hands, telling her that her behavior would anger God because it was sinful, and prohibiting her from engaging in it. In fact, Alicia had placed gloves on Jenna's hands at night and had also tied her hands on occasion so that she wouldn't touch herself. Alicia volunteered that Jenna often had frequent urinary tract infections, but that the family pediatrician had thought they were related to bubble baths, which Alicia had stopped promptly at the physician's suggestion.

When we talked about the relationship between Jenna and her brother, Roberto, Alicia noted that there was some "sibling rivalry," which she described as "Jenna doesn't like us to give him attention; she wants us to notice her only!" When I asked how Alicia and James responded to Jenna's need for attention or her jealousy when Roberto got attention, Alicia said that they talked to her about loving both children, and usually divided the children between the two of them, giving them both individual time. Alicia said that at other times, Jenna was perfectly wonderful to her little brother, "patient and loving." As Alicia was walking out of this assessment session, she "remembered" that Jenna had once pulled Roberto's pants off and begun pinching his penis. She said that on that occasion she had slapped Jenna's hand and punished her (no dinner that night).

Both children slept in the same room when Alicia first came for assessment, but she was quick to say that they were preparing a more "feminine room" for Jenna; this was almost ready for her, and they were moving Roberto into Phillip's room. Alicia told me that Phillip was a "brilliant student," who had skipped two grades and would be going off to college soon. She described Phillip as a "good student and role model" for his younger cousins—a child who was extremely close to his father and to God. Phillip had never given the family any trouble, had dated the same girl for 2 years, and was very active in the youth program of their church. Alicia and James felt "blessed" by Phillip. When I asked what it had been like for him to have these two young children move into his home when he was only 10, Alicia noted that Phillip was very helpful to her and James in caring for the youngsters, but that he was very devoted to soccer when he was younger, and later replaced that intense interest with studying and reading. She described him as "quiet as a mouse, usually in his room on his Internet, studying, or with his girlfriend at her house." It seemed that Phillip had been only peripherally involved with Jenna and Roberto.

I gave Alicia some information about what to do about Jenna's masturbatory behavior, and I commended her for having made efforts to guide the child in the past. I told her that although she had come up with a few good ideas, there were other ideas that might work as well or better, and not cause other problems (e.g., tying Jenna's hands might scare the child and could cause risk if she had to get out of her bed). Alicia was receptive to my feedback in her way. She was definite in her belief that touching oneself was a sin, however, and was not willing to take a more relaxed approach to this. My hope was that as she began attending the Boundary Project group for parents/caregivers, she might begin to soften her responses, but I was also aware that religious rules often provide an external control that makes sense to caregivers and their children. I believe that religious rules can serve as an important foundation to help children make good choices, but will need to be supplemented by other guidance at times—especially when children are acting out their own traumas and may not be in a position to choose their behaviors, because they are fueled by emotional distress or overwhelming affect associated with past unresolved events.

I described the Boundary Project program to Alicia, and she was relieved to hear that she could have her husband come half of the time. Alicia's family schedule was very demanding, and adding one more thing would be difficult. I emphasized with Alicia that after the assessment I would know what to recommend, but that our assessment was designed to identify how children were doing, what was going on with their thinking and behavior, and what their individual needs were. I also told Alicia that how family members responded—their ideas, their willingness to help us help their children—were part of the things we looked at to decide what was needed.

I commended Alicia on following up on this referral, on being interested and invested in Jenna and Roberto, and on her receptivity to our discussion and the guidelines I was offering. She agreed to 24/7 supervision of Jenna, which would be shared by herself, her husband, and even Phillip when he was available. She had been aware that Jenna showed some "flirtatiousness" with Phillip and had asked him early to be cautious in all contacts with her—something Jenna perceived as "he doesn't like me." Alicia's ability to think ahead that Jenna's relationship with Phillip could be challenging was another good sign of her ability to take a proactive and preventive stance.

Alicia was willing to try some other ways of addressing Alicia's masturbatory behaviors. She had already separated the children at night and was expediting the completion of Jenna's new room. This would allow each child to have a separate room (Roberto's would be his alone once Phillip left for college), and at the same time would attend to Jenna's need to feel special to Alicia and James (they had been working with her on decorating her room and had bought her the canopy bed of her dreams).

Initial Assessment Impressions

Jenna was initially very lukewarm about assessment and the prospect of therapy. She felt that she was "in trouble" with her family, and she viewed assessment and therapy as a kind of punishment for wrongdoing. She was defiant with me, threw things around the room, and told me I was "old enough to be retired" (a very observant and smart thing to notice). I agreed with her and smiled as she kept asking how old I was. I used a nondirective approach with her initially, except when I asked her what she had been told about coming to therapy. We had a very interesting initial conversation, which I believe went a long way toward setting a more positive context for our work.

> JENNA: My mom [i.e., Alicia] thinks that I'm weird and gross, and she says you think that too!
>
> THERAPIST: Hmmm. I don't remember anybody using the words "weird" and "gross."
>
> JENNA: Well, what did my mom say?
>
> THERAPIST: I will be happy to share that with you, but first I want to understand what your mom told you about coming here.
>
> JENNA: She told me that I was doing bad things and that you thought they were bad things.
>
> THERAPIST: Do you know what she was talking about?
>
> JENNA: You know . . .
>
> THERAPIST: Well, I'm not really sure what you mean by "bad things."
>
> JENNA: Bad things when I touch my parts, down there, or when I touch my brother's weenie.
>
> THERAPIST: I think that it's important to learn that private parts belong just to you, and it's not OK to touch other people's private parts.
>
> JENNA: I know. I don't know what makes me bad.
>
> THERAPIST: Well, I didn't say you were "bad." I said it was important to not touch other people's private parts.
>
> JENNA: I know, I know.
>
> THERAPIST: So did your mom tell you what my job is?
>
> JENNA: No.
>
> THERAPIST: My job is to get to know you, get to know what you like to do, how things are going for you.
>
> JENNA: And then what?
>
> THERAPIST: And then to figure out how to help you, so that you know what to do when you get thoughts or ideas about touching private parts.
>
> JENNA: OK, OK, I don't want to talk about this any more.

THERAPIST: And we don't have to, right now. I'd like us to get to know each other a little. But later on, I will ask you to either show me or talk to me about this problem behavior.

JENNA: It's not a problem to me!

THERAPIST: It's not?

JENNA: No . . . except I get in trouble with my mom and dad.

THERAPIST: Oh, so it is a problem to you, because you get in trouble with your parents.

JENNA: Yeah, OK, I want to play now.

THERAPIST: OK, we can play. This is your time for picking out what you'd like to do or say in here."

JENNA: Let's play Mankala. I'll beat your butt!

THERAPIST: You sound confident that you can win. OK, let's play Mankala.

And this is probably the best example of how we worked. Jenna was initially provocative and defiant, but this protesting usually gave way to compliance and participation. She was a very energetic, spirited, impulsive child, with a short attention span. She was also clearly ambivalent about interacting with others—perhaps because she was expecting to be seen as bad, to get in trouble, or to have someone control her behaviors. The more we interacted, the more evident it became to her that I respected her choices, that I would not push her, and that I would follow her pace. Sometimes she wanted to cooperate; sometimes she did not. Sometimes she wanted to participate in an activity; sometimes she did not. Her sessions reflected whether she had had a good or bad day at school, and she expressed herself very clearly. She became comfortable enough to ask for the Affective Scaling Sheets. She liked deciding which feeling she felt before and after our sessions (see Form 5.2) and used the Body Thermometer when her feelings were more intense (see Form 5.3). Because she was able to show her emotions so well, I began to comment on how well she got her point across. Slowly but surely, she developed pride about how well she showed her feelings and how well this enabled me to guess them. We established a routine of her exaggerating physical manifestations of an emotion, and my describing what she was doing and guessing. I also began asking her to "rate the feeling" she was having on a scale of 1 to 5, and on occasion, I would ask her to show me the feeling and take it up or down a notch. This was a playful interaction that had therapeutic benefit, in that it expanded her emotional language and gave her a sense of mastery. One day when Jenna was playing the "feeling game," and showing me how frustrated she felt with her teacher (whom Jenna described as "picking on her"), I asked her to do something else.

THERAPIST: . . . I see, so the more she asked you to slow down and write your name more carefully, the more frustrated you got!

JENNA: Why does it have to be at her speed? I like to write fast. I can write faster than everybody.

THERAPIST: So you're really confident that you can write faster than anybody!

JENNA: I really can. I've had contests with some of the kids in the class.

THERAPIST: No kidding! A write-faster-than everybody contest— that sounds like fun!

JENNA: Well, it is, and I beat everybody all the time!

THERAPIST: Awesome, but sounds like the teacher likes you to slow it down.

JENNA: I don't care! She's always picking on me.

THERAPIST: Oh, so you think she's picking on you.

JENNA: She is. She's mean!

THERAPIST: And you feel frustrated and angry, right?

JENNA: Yeah, like this . . . (*Jenna bends her head down, frowns, and flexes her arms forward, making a scary-looking posture.*)

THERAPIST: Wowza! You look really angry.

JENNA: Gggggggggggrrrrrrrrrrrrrr!

THERAPIST: Hey, I have an idea. Think for a minute. What is the opposite of feeling frustrated and angry?

JENNA: I don't know.

THERAPIST: Just think for a minute. What would be the opposite of that?

JENNA: (*Is pensive for a few minutes and really seems to consider this.*) I guess it would be like this. (*Jenna puts her hands in front of her as if praying, and puts an angelic smile on her face, relaxing her body.*)

THERAPIST: Oh, this looks quite different from angry and frustrated. Hold on, hold on, let me take another look and I'll rate it.

JENNA: OK! (*Jenna rearranges her stance, tilts her head, keeps her hands together, points upward, and places a nice smile on her face.*)

THERAPIST: I'm gonna say that's content and peaceful at a 5!

JENNA: Close, a 4+!

THERAPIST: Awesome, I came really close.

JENNA: Yeah, close but no banana.

THERAPIST: You were great at showing the opposite of the other feeling you were having. It's good to know what the opposite feelings are and what they look like.

JENNA: Let me show you the opposite of this one!

THERAPIST: Oh, I see that angry, frustrated body again. But wait, I'm noticing there's a little change. It doesn't look so, so angry . . . let me guess, let me guess. I think this is frustrated and angry at a 2.

JENNA: Yeah, that's it!

THERAPIST: I got it perfectly right? All right! That doesn't always happen to me, but you're really good at showing things.

JENNA: Yep, I got lots of things I'm good at.

THERAPIST: You know what I was thinking, Jenna? (*She looks up.*) You've shown your teacher how fast a writer you are. Maybe you can teach her how slow a writer you can be.

JENNA: (*Looks down and does not respond.*)

THERAPIST: Well, I mean, if you think you can master the opposite of writing fast, the art of the tortoise, writing slow . . . that might be a big challenge to someone who's perfected the art of writing fast.

JENNA: I can do it!

THERAPIST: I think you just might, because you're really good at opposites!

Jenna began practicing writing slowly that day in the session. At the next session, she reported with some sense of mastery that her teacher was shocked that she didn't have to correct her for doing things too fast!

Jenna had the uncanny ability to turn many things into opportunities for mastery and growth.

Much of Jenna's early, nondirective artwork is present only in my memory. She did not want me to take photos of it because she did not feel that anything she did was "good enough." She often took her art-work home with her, where she crumpled it or tore it up, or she hid it somewhere in the home. Alicia told me that Jenna kept many things under her mattress, including several things she had apparently taken from my office. When I learned about the fact that she was taking things from the office, I asked her not to do so, because they wouldn't be there for her or other children to play with when she or they were in my office. I also told her that since she was good at hiding and taking things, this would require me to watch her a little more closely. Jenna was always trying to bend or break rules. For example, children in our office often take a snack from a basket in the back of the office. Jenna had seen other children get snacks, and she asked if she could do the same. I told her she could, so every time she came we went to the back. Sometimes she ran ahead of me, and every time we looked at the snack basket, she literally begged for more than one snack. I held to a firm limit, but sometimes when she ran ahead, she grabbed a second snack and held one under the other. Eventually we ended up having to do a "search" before she left, because she consistently tried to sneak out a second snack. My inter-pretation of this was that she was trying to verify, over and over, that I would not change the rule. For Jenna, a firm rule was very important, and the searching also became our closing ritual. It appeared that she liked the little extra attention that she got from me, and enjoyed the game she initiated with me about searching. It was reminiscent of a game one might play with a developmentally younger child, such as "hide and seek" or "peek-a-boo."

I invited Jenna to participate in several play-based activities, and her participation wavered with her moods. As mentioned earlier, I quickly learned that Jenna's moods fluctuated greatly, primarily depending on whether she had gotten in trouble at school or at home. It turned out that Jenna had a great deal of impulsive behavior; it also became appar-ent that social interactions elicited a lot of anxiety, that she struggled greatly with her self-image, that kids teased her about not living with her "real" mother and father, and that she still harbored insecurities about whether her placement with her aunt and uncle was permanent. During the assessment, she confided to me that "I'm always in trouble. My brain is talking to me all the time. I think I must be bad, like . . . " Eventually she told me that she thought her mother had been "bad" all her life, and that she was probably going to be just like her. These very basic ideas filled her with anxiety and distress, and she tended to act these emotions out, unaware of how to quiet them or the negative thoughts that gave rise to them. Systemically, and paradoxically, Alicia's desire to wait to adopt Jenna and Roberto (in order to give her sister a chance to reha-bilitate herself) had had a confusing impact on Jenna, who felt unstable and unwanted by either her mother or her aunt (whom she now called "Mom").

The assessment proceeded well as far as my getting to know Jenna and establishing a therapeutic relationship with her. However, in regard to her participating fully in assessment activities, or speaking more directly about her touching problems, she remained hesitant and unavailable. I learned a lot about many of the issues that were probably contributing to her acting out—but, more important, I learned about Jenna and some of the ways that her early experiences had shaped some of her expectations, some of her insecurities, and some of the life ques-tions that needed clarity (e.g., "Where do I belong? Am I lovable? Who is my mother? What happens if I'm 'too bad'?")

Structured Assessment Tasks

Drawing Tasks

Certain aspects of the more structured assessment tasks stood out. The most memorable thing about Jenna's self-portrait, for example, was that it was so small and drawn in such light pencil lines that it was barely visible. It had no ground line, and as a matter of fact, it lacked any details. A very small, almost invisible figure appeared as if floating on the page; the rest of the page was empty. Interestingly, the mouth included large teeth, and there were multiple erasures on the lower part of her body. When teeth are included in drawings by children Jenna's age, they can be suggestive of anger or rage. The erasures on the bottom part of her body could suggest some discomfort with drawing that part of her body.

When Jenna made an ambivalent attempt at the K-F-D (for which the directive is "Draw a picture of you and your family doing some-thing together"), she did include a ground line, a house, and herself. The self-depiction looked more substantial than the one in the self-portrait (darker lines, more defined dress, no teeth), and she portrayed herself with her left hand holding on to Alicia's hand and her right hand holding on to Roberto's hand. Roberto was holding on to Phillip, who had his father's hand. It was particularly interesting that Jenna drew another head on top of her own and then erased it. She put that second circle above her own head after she made her own figure and almost as an afterthought, when she sat back and looked at her picture with me. "Oops," she said and made the circle, but then erased it. I wondered what her change had been, and she said, "Never mind." I didn't push her on this and simply described what I had seen: "When you were looking at your picture, you said, 'Oops,' and then made a circle on top of your head. Then you erased it and left it erased. Looked to me like you remembered something you wanted to include and then did so." She did not respond. My interpretation (which I kept to myself) was that Jenna viewed her mother as a ghost or an angel, and she had acknowledged that fact. Jenna felt her mother's presence, and maybe she missed her or hoped for her to return, or maybe she simply knew that Glenda would always be an unreachable figure in her life.

Sand Therapy

Jenna also liked to play in the sand tray, and her style of working was predictable and consistent. She would ask first for water to wet the sand, and although in her first efforts she "flooded" the sand (which made any construction impossible), after three or four attempts she began to wet the sand enough that she could construct very high mountain peaks—or at least that was what they looked like to me. She took great care to gather and mold the sand in such a way that each mountain was thick at the bottom and rose to a much thinner, pointed peak. She used her whole body to do this, often getting wet sand on her arms, her elbows, and the front of her shirt. I learned to put a round plastic rug under the sand tray when she came to her sessions. She took great pleasure in making each peak high and using every grain of sand that was available to her. She derived a sense of mastery from making this tall peak, as evidenced by her behavior after she finished: She wanted me to take multiple pictures from many angles, especially those pictures that showed how far over the boundary of the tray the peak had emerged.

Jenna never did any other shapes in the sand, but she eventually added some animals (see Figure 9.1). One tray in particular had two sheep with a "touching problem," as well as a mother and child pig and a large furnace. She was once able to do a tray in response to a directive

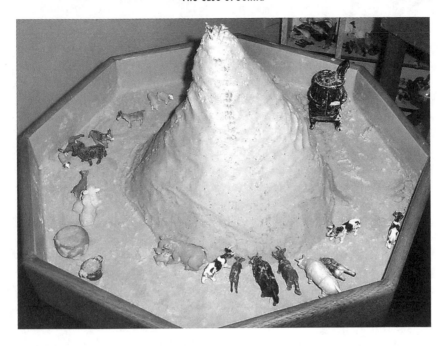

FIGURE 9.1. Jenna's sand tray: "I can build high to the sky and beyond."

(i.e., "Show me the touching problem in the tray"); this tray did not include a large peak.

TREATMENT PLAN, GOALS, AND PROCESS

Jenna did not complete any other structured assessment activities. However, I felt that I was able to develop a treatment plan based on the assessment, which would include individual therapy with me to advance specific goals not related to her sexual behavior problems. I also referred Jenna and her parents to the Boundary Project (see Chapter Six) for participation in the parallel group therapy process. Alicia and James agreed enthusiastically to attend, and said that they would come together to as many scheduled group sessions as their work schedules would permit.

My individual work with Jenna focused on the larger picture and a very specific goal: to clarify Jenna's family situation, especially her current and future placement. She had an insecure attachment to both mother figures—Glenda, her birth mother, and Alicia, the biological aunt who would soon be her adoptive mother. My goal was to help the family clarify to Jenna what was going on in regard to Glenda, the termination of Glenda's parental rights, and the adoption by Alicia and James. In addition, it would be important for Alicia to know what to expect about future contact with her birth mother—where she lived, whether she could or could not contact her, and whether she would see her again.

A secondary goal was to create a historical narrative with Jenna, so that her perceptions of prior experiences and relationships could be addressed. Although Jenna had not reported specific memories of either observing or experiencing sexual abuse, there was reason to believe that something might have happened to Jenna during one of those times when she was with her birth mother and out of contact with Alicia. Since Alicia had maintained ongoing contact with her sister and had many opportunities to talk to her during her sober moments, Alicia suspected that Glenda's lifestyle was incredibly unpredictable and unsafe, although Glenda had a consistent style of denying and covering up wrongdoing.

Last, I was very interested in assisting Jenna to find new ways of thinking of herself, more positive self-talking, and a more balanced view of her strengths and weaknesses. This goal was closely linked to helping Jenna establish a consistent relationship with a peer—something she had been unable to do on her own. Although the peer group in the Boundary Project allowed for some social contact, the setting did not seem to help much; the fact that there were six other girls in the group, all vying for attention, activated intense reactions for Jenna. She also seemed to feel left out, and the other girls seemed to gravitate more toward each other. Indeed, Jenna seemed to contribute to replicating in the group some of the social dynamics she was experiencing in her school, and because the focus of this group was on reducing sexual behavior problems, other strategies for enhancing group dynamics were not prioritized. However, as Alicia and I were able to plan a more gradual approach (supervised play dates, like those arranged for much younger children), Jenna was able to reap the benefits of a successful friendship with a distant cousin her age and gender.

As just noted , Jenna's Boundary Project group focused specifically on sexual behavior problems, while she and I did collateral work individually. Although specific goals of the Boundary Project are listed elsewhere (see Chapter Six), the following goals were particularly relevant for Jenna and her family:

1. Learning about physical boundaries, and teaching siblings and parents these principles.
2. Learning about affective expression, particularly the Color Your Feelings technique, and having family members use this and share it with each other.
3. Helping Jenna understand the origins of her problem thoughts and behaviors, particularly where the "touching ideas" came from.
4. Finally, having Jenna and her brother understand the types of touch that were and were not appropriate between them, and what to do when inappropriate thoughts entered their minds.

Specifically, I used hula hoops to explain to Jenna that we all have "private space" that belongs to us alone, and that we don't go into other's private spaces, and they don't go into ours. Jenna made her understanding gloriously clear when she announced loudly, "And, you don't go into other people's private parts either!" Alicia, James, and I commended her for this insight, which she seemed to have truly integrated. The Boundary Project provided her with useful information about victimization; her own victimization work was done in individual therapy.

Jenna remained in individual therapy for almost a year. During that time, she slowly confided that one of her mother's boyfriends, Gustavo, had put his fingers inside her vagina and rectum while her mother lay asleep in the same bed. Gustavo had also threatened to hurt her and to throw her out of the house if she told her mother. Finally, Jenna described that Gustavo would grab her face and turn it toward him as he had sex with her mother, who was usually asleep. From her description and the sense of fear and confusion she felt, it was clear that Jenna had been traumatized by this man, and that she had escaped even greater harm when (as she described it) the police had come and arrested him one night and she never saw him again. Jenna was able eventually to process her thoughts and feelings about these incidents; as she did so, she looked visibly relieved to be telling someone about what had occurred and what she had survived. When she processed this and reclaimed her sense of personal power, she wanted to tell Alicia and found great comfort in her arms. Of particular value to this child was drawing a picture of Gustavo, then taking a thick black marker and covering his face up completely. "I sometimes see those eyes staring at me, but now I just wipe them out!" Jenna would then take the picture, make a paper ball of it, and throw it in the trash.

Jenna developed a real affinity for most art-based activities. The Color Your Feelings technique (see Chapter Four and Form 4.2) was a big hit with this family, and one member would frequently pull out a gingerbread person and ask other family members to show their feelings by using colors. Jenna would always instruct Roberto, "If you have a lotta, lotta, lotta one feeling, then you color that one all over!" This simple art activity captured their imagination and facilitated much self-disclosure and discussion.

Many of our family therapy sessions focused on the issue of adoption. This family chose to emphasize that Jenna and Roberto were special gifts to them from God, and that God had chosen them all to be a family. When Jenna asked why God hadn't taken good care of their mother, Glenda, Alicia reassured her and Roberto that God would never abandon Glenda, but that Glenda had to *"dar de su parte"* (translation: "put in her part"), and that God would do the rest. James and Alicia had also been wise to inform their children about the dangers of drugs, the difficulty of struggling with addiction, and the suffering this painful disease causes for many people. Jenna found some comfort in thinking of her mother as "sick" and unable to care for them because of her illness.

The family expressed great joy at becoming a "permanent" family. One of our last sessions involved having James and Alicia read the children a book called *The Invisible String* (Karst, 2000), which talks about the ties binding us to people who may not be physically present, but who love us and whom we love. This certainly applied in Glenda's case: She had been unable to provide for her children, and had lost many a fight against her addiction, but always seemed concerned with making sure someone was available to help and provide for the children. Glenda was unable to attend a "goodbye session" with her children, due to a recent incarceration on drug possession charges; however, she sent them a card telling them to listen to their new parents, Alicia and James, and encouraging them to keep doing well in school. Jenna and Roberto took her words to heart. Alicia and James also spoke of Roberto's and Jenna's fathers, stating that they also had been unable to provide for them and saying they would always be in their prayers. Jenna and I had discussed her ideas about her biological father, what he would look like, and what he would be like. Jenna had stated that she could not even imagine him, but hoped that if she had known him and had to live with him, she hoped he would be "just like my real dad, James." Both Roberto and Jenna seemed to have a meaningful attachment to James, who seemed to be the glue that held the family together. In his quiet and humble way, he was a reliable and gentle father figure and provided the children with the empathic care and consistent presence they required to trust and respect him fully.

SUMMARY AND CONCLUSIONS

Jenna, a Hispanic 7-year-old, was an attractive, funny, energetic child with a difficult history—including a mother with chronic problems of drug addiction; a father she had never known, who caused feelings of unresolved loss; placement with her aunt and uncle, which generated ambivalent responses in Jenna; removal into foster care prior to going to her aunt and uncle's home; and exposure to inappropriate sexual behaviors by adults, as well as physical and sexual abuse and neglect. The fact that Jenna's mother had drifted in and out of her life had confused and worried Jenna, who exhibited many of the symptoms associated with children of alcoholic/addicted parents, including focused attention on her mother's care.

Jenna's soon-to-be adoptive parents (her biological aunt and the aunt's husband) had taken voluntary custody of Jenna and her brother, but they had only recently formalized plans to adopt the children. Jenna's birth mother, Glenda, lived in constant turmoil but had the strength and good sense to turn to her older sister, Alicia, to help her with her children.

The concerns about Jenna at the time of her referral included inappropriate sexual behaviors toward her younger brother, defiant and dysregulated behaviors, and emotionality. It is interesting to note that these symptoms are some of the observable signs of posttraumatic stress disorder, and this child appeared to have suffered both generic and specific traumas throughout her young life. In addition, Alicia and her husband, James, expressed concern about Jenna's constant interest in Glenda (when she would return to live with her, etc.). In cases like Jenna's, the sexual behavior problems are often the manifestations of other concerns, and comprehensive assessments usually reveal a host of areas that must be addressed in treatment.

Alicia and her husband were very invested in these young children (which made our eventual job much easier) and had begun adoption proceedings in spite of Glenda's anemic protests. They had not, however, told the children, wanting to wait until the court made a final decision.

Child protective services personnel were eventually called in and encouraged Alicia and James to formalize the children's placement. In their new home, the children experienced consistent and empathic care, interrupted only by erratic visits from Glenda as well as brief removals into her care. Alicia finally set very firm limits and decided to fight her sister for the right to adopt her children and provide a consistent and loving environment for them.

Jenna's sexual acting out (the proximal cause of the child protective services referral) seemed precipitated by posttraumatic memories of abuse, which seemed to emerge in relationship to the impending court proceedings regarding termination of Glenda's parental rights and adoption by Alicia and James. She was insecurely attached to her birth mother and had developed great concern for her, often worrying about how much she was eating or if she was sleeping properly. She seemed agitated when her aunt was unable to tell her where her mother was living, but eventually she understood that her mother had a sickness and needed help from the doctors to get well enough to take good care of herself. Alicia communicated clearly to Jenna that Glenda understood that she could not take good care of her children, and had asked her to parent them and give them the home she could not provide. Jenna found some comfort in knowing that her mother wanted her to be happy with her new parents, and that when Glenda was healthy she could become a part of her life again, but that this would not change the fact that she was now in her permanent home. Paradoxically, Jenna's learning that her mother would no longer be able to come and take her and Roberto away seemed to lessen many of her fears and concerns; both her sleeping and eating habits seemed to normalize at this point including some of her hoarding behaviors. (I guessed that she might be saving food for her mother.)

Jenna's sexual behavior problems were addressed easily once these other contextual issues were addressed. As she became able to discuss some of the sexual situations she had seen and experienced between her mother and the mother's boyfriends (she drew repeated pictures of two nude persons on a bed), some of her anxiety decreased. She was able to verbalize that one boyfriend, Gustavo, had touched her privates, and that she didn't like it and cried. When I told her that it wasn't OK for anyone to touch her private parts, she said in a meek voice, "And I can't touch nobody's either." I agreed that this was true. I told Jenna that adults (like Gustavo) know that what they are doing is wrong, and they go ahead and do the wrong thing anyway. "He had a problem in his thinking and doing. It was wrong of him to touch your privates!" She liked that phrase and made it into a song that she often sang in my office.

As emphasized throughout this chapter, Jenna was very resilient and managed to turn many situations into mastery opportunities. Her recovery was also greatly enhanced by having a strong adoptive family, grounded in spiritual faith and practice, with a strong commitment to her and her brother. Jenna finally achieved a secure base, loving parents, and a sense of predictability and consistency. These factors held great promise for her future.

CHAPTER TEN

The Case of Lorenzo

REFERRAL INFORMATION

Lorenzo was 11 years old when I (E. G.) first met him. He had arrived from El Salvador 6 months earlier, after living with his paternal grandparents for most of his life, ever since his father and mother had come to the United States when Lorenzo was 2 years old. Since that time, Lorenzo's mother and father had talked to him from time to time, sent money home for his care, and always stayed true to their expressed goal of bringing him to join them when they could afford to do so. Lorenzo was referred to me for sexually abusing his 6-year-old sister, Anna Maria, almost from the day he arrived. Anna Maria reported the sexual abuse to her mother, who told her son to stop "bothering" Anna Maria. Later, Anna Maria told her guidance counselor at school, who reported the case to child protective services. Since that time, Anna Maria had been referred for "individual victim therapy," the family was receiving home-based services, and the investigators had referred Lorenzo for therapy. Because Lorenzo was not a caregiver to his sister, and the parents were always in the home while Lorenzo was molesting Anna Maria, he was not removed from the home. However, the parents were told in no uncertain terms that they had to follow up on specialized therapy for "young sex offenders," and the county allocated funds to pay for therapy services.

PSYCHOSOCIAL BACKGROUND

Lorenzo's parents, José and Hilda, had come from El Salvador with high hopes of saving themselves and their families from a life with dead ends, no resources, and a lack of alternatives. They had watched their own parents struggle with poverty—working long, hard days in the fields, and coming home to make limited food stretch to feed many mouths. They had both seen their fathers work from sundown to sunrise, drink themselves to sleep, exhibit bouts of violence, disappear for periods of time, and get old and sickly before their time. Hilda's parents had died when she was very young, in a bus accident during a flood. José's parents were debilitated by ill health, alcoholism, and pessimism. José and Hilda knew that leaving Lorenzo behind was their only option, but they also knew that his elderly grandparents would be ill prepared to supervise, nurture, or educate him. The only driving force for them was "getting ahead" in a land they perceived to have many opportunities.

Of course, when they arrived in the United States, they encountered many problems they had not anticipated: Jobs were very hard to get without immigration papers; there was tremendous competition for each and every job; and wages were low, while costs for rent, food, and transportation were high. In order to avoid having more children, which could divert them from working long hours and multiple jobs, they stopped sleeping together, choosing instead to work whatever shifts and whatever jobs would pay something. Hilda cleaned houses, washed dishes, swept sidewalks, and on occasion, took care of the infants of some of her friends who either had more regular work or could count on her to watch the children while they got impromptu day jobs. José went out early each morning to a street corner where 20–30 men gathered, available to work anywhere, for any wage. Some days he was fortunate enough to get picked up for work, and he tried hard to please his temporary bosses. Other days he hung around the streets, begging for money, which he would then spend on alcohol. Sometimes he stayed out all night sleeping in the streets, because he was ashamed to go home without funds.

A number of years later, Hilda became pregnant by another man and had her daughter, Anna Maria. She convinced José that Anna Maria was his child; at the time of intake, Hilda was still guarding this secret, fearing for her life if she told. The child seemed to bring them together and appease some of their sadness over Lorenzo's absence, and the fact that she was a little girl seemed to motivate José to curb his drinking, to keep working hard when he could, and to find further employment. Up to this point, they had shared a rented room with another couple. When Anna Maria was born, they asked the other couple to leave, and the three of them shared the large room. Hilda had saved quite a nest egg, which she guarded closely, afraid her husband would "drink it away." José had also met some employers who liked his stamina and ability to learn quickly, so he started getting more regular pay. The parents were able to send more money for Lorenzo's care, not knowing that all the funds they were sacrificing so much to earn were funding Lorenzo's grandfather's alcoholism and gambling.

Once Anna Maria entered the school system, the guidance counselor noticed her torn clothing and apparent hunger. Anna Maria's counselor called in a social worker and got Hilda qualified to get general assistance from the county department of family services. Slowly but surely, the family's situation improved, and Hilda learned to negotiate her way around the system. José, on the other hand, led a more insulated life—working hard when he could, but sleeping and drinking when work was not found. They did, however, have another child when Anna Maria was about 4 years old, and they described this child, Pedro, as a "good boy." José and Hilda continued to work hard to reach their goal of having their oldest son join them, and were eventually able to rent a two-bedroom apartment. Finally, when Lorenzo turned 11, friends from El Salvador picked him up and brought him across the border to his parents.

Lorenzo was a smart and resourceful child who had experienced great trauma in his life. His grandfather had taken him out into the streets at an early age, and he had seen drug use, prostitution, gambling, and violence. He hung out with much older boys, and also learned to drink and smoke marijuana; however, he was slight in build and not very threatening-looking, so the others tended to leave him alone, and some of his older friends watched out for him. Lorenzo was also an attractive boy who elicited the attention of many adult males. Eventually, Lorenzo's grandfather found that he could earn good money by selling Lorenzo to men who wanted oral sex from him. Even later in our treatment, Lorenzo was unable or unwilling to talk about his street experiences, but it was clear that he had experienced multiple traumatic events that confused and scared him. Lorenzo seemed to want me to think that he was a "tough guy" who could take care of himself pretty well. According to Lorenzo, at first his grandfather would get most of the money; later Lorenzo sought out his own customers and stopped giving his grandfather a cut of his earnings. One of the reasons he was ambivalent when his parents sent for him was that he was getting used to earning good money as a very young and popular male prostitute.

When Lorenzo arrived in the United States, he was unhappy to be uprooted. He looked around with surprise at his parents' modest, now crowded apartment, and was not able to understand that the two Americanized children with whom he now shared it were his siblings. He was particularly disdainful to his sister, Anna Maria, whom he found "strange and annoying." The fact that she mostly spoke in English really bothered him, and he didn't like how clean her clothes were or the fact that she was a little overweight. He started teasing her almost immediately, and Anna Maria became distressed, because up to that moment her parents had treated her with kindness. In fact, she was a little "spoiled," according to her mother.

Hilda and José bent over backward to allow Lorenzo to adapt; their efforts were motivated by guilt that they had left him behind for so long. Lorenzo began to confide in his father about his life, and José was furious that the money he had earned and sent his father had gone mostly toward supporting his father's bad street habits. Lorenzo also shared with José that his grandfather had gotten money by selling him to men for oral sex, and José shared that the same things had happened to him as a child. He encouraged Lorenzo to "forget about his life in El Salvador," the same way he had. He assured Lorenzo that things would be different for him here.

Hilda kept encouraging Anna Maria to seek out her brother, to show him the playground nearby, and to be extra nice to him. Lorenzo, however, got more and more irritated when he was around her. He liked his little brother better, and especially liked earning dollars to take care of him. Hilda never left Lorenzo alone with Anna Maria, sensing his rancor toward her. She did, however, leave Lorenzo to take care of Pedro, and Lorenzo seemed very patient and sweet with him. When I remarked to the mother that Pedro was precisely the same age as Lorenzo had been when she and her husband had left him in the care of his paternal grandparents, Hilda cried, saying that she had not noticed the coincidence.

José and Hilda were shocked and pained to hear that Lorenzo had made sexual advances toward Anna Maria, and at first they insisted that Anna Maria had innocently misinterpreted what must have been brotherly affection. When Anna Maria first talked to her mother, Hilda hushed her and told her she would speak to Lorenzo. What she actually said to Lorenzo was this: "Sweetie, your sister is feeling a little shy when you get close to her. Please don't get too close to her, OK?" Lorenzo agreed to that, but behind his mother's back he went to Anna Maria and told her that he would kill her if she said another word to her parents about whatever he chose to do with her. "You have no rights in this house any more. You are no one, and I can do what I want. Don't let me catch you talking to them again, or else!" he said, lifting his wrist. Anna Maria was smart enough to know that her brother meant business, and also smart enough to know her parents were not able to help her—so after a week, she talked to the school guidance counselor, whom she trusted. At this point, child protective services became involved.

The referral was somewhat unclear to me initially, since the parents told me, "Something happened. We're not sure what, and we don't really want to know. We just want Lorenzo to stay with us, and we don't want him to go to jail." The intake session with the parents revealed two reasons for their hesitancy to know details about the sexual abuse: (1) a reluctance to think that an 11-year-old could do much physical damage to his sister (particularly since both children were so small); and (2) their conviction that Anna Maria was still a virgin, because a pediatrician had told them so (the pediatrician had done a cursory external exam of her and declared her virginal, which of course was a great relief to the parents). Given their belief that Anna Maria's virginity was intact, José and Hilda felt certain that "nothing too bad had happened, thank the Lord." José and Hilda never inquired about the emotional impact of being sexually abused and threatened by her brother, and they asked few questions about how to help her. Like many Hispanic parents in their situation, they wanted both children to forget what had happened and to move on. Hilda also prayed for her daughter and son, and put things in God's hands. She was a woman who found comfort in her religious activities, and this was a resource I knew would become useful in her recovery.

After the parents explained why they had been referred (albeit in a constricted manner), I explained our services to them. Lorenzo would have an assessment, during which we would gauge how willing he was to talk honestly about what had happened, and how amenable he was to receiving help. Anna Maria would be referred to her own individual therapist, to gauge the extent of her abuse and to identify and assist her with whatever impact this short-lived sexual abuse had had on her. Her therapist eventually gave Anna Maria considerable positive feedback for telling not only once, to her mother, but twice; for knowing that this behavior was not appropriate; and for allowing us to help her and her brother. ("I don't know him very well," Anna Maria told this therapist. "He grew up in our old country.")

Parents agreed to our therapy schedule and accepted home-based services as well. There was close collaboration between the children's clinicians and the home-based program, to ensure appropriate supervision, monitoring, and safety. Given that Lorenzo had remained in his parents' care, it was critical to decrease their denial and increase their supervision immediately. The child protective services worker visited the home and told the parents in no uncertain terms that if anything else happened, even if Lorenzo "looked at Anna Maria sideways," he would be removed to a juvenile facility. This put the fear of God in the parents, who moved Anna Maria into their room; took Lorenzo out of Pedro's room (at the advice of the social worker); and put Lorenzo in the living room, alone, and away from his siblings. All rooms got locks, and the parents also agreed to put bells on the door so that they could hear when the children were coming or going. Most important, the child protective services worker told Lorenzo (in front of his parents) that his threats to his sister would not be tolerated. José and Hilda implored Lorenzo to follow all the rules and avoid ruining their efforts to have him be part of their family *"por fin"* ("finally"). They begged him to follow all directives, so that he could continue to stay in this country and avoid deportation to a life full of suffering and dead ends. Information about sibling abuse was translated into Spanish and provided to the parents (see Form 10.1 for the English version).

Because it was so urgent to decrease the parents' denial, we initially met with Lorenzo twice a week. Surprisingly, Lorenzo was only noncompliant during the first session! After that, he seemed to thrive on the focused attention he received. The assessment process proceeded well, as described below, and after each session we talked to the parents about what had been discussed. This type of transparency was very important to decrease parental denial, to discourage family secrecy, and to strengthen the weak and unformed parent–child connection.

Hilda continued with her various jobs while José opted to stay home more often, sometimes working the overnight shift. In addition, after we started meeting in June, Lorenzo was referred to English as a Second Language classes in summer school to give him a head start on learning English, since he would be entering school in the fall. Because he had received no formal education in "the old country," it was unclear what grade placement would be made. However, it seemed that Lorenzo was streetwise, intuitive, and capable of learning. Lorenzo did well in summer school, tested at about second-grade reading level in Spanish, and was assessed to enter the fourth grade. Given his small stature, when he entered school other children did not tease him for being younger, and he met other children who were struggling to learn English.

ASSESSMENT PROCESS

Initial Assessment Impressions

As mentioned earlier, Lorenzo was minimally resistant to the assessment process. Mostly he seemed like a neglected child, eager to please, and desirous of positive attention and nurturing. He began opening up early, and the more he spoke about his early life, the bleaker the picture became. Lorenzo seemed to be a highly resilient child who had overcome tremendous adverse experiences in his life and somehow managed not only to survive, but to fend for himself. It's hard to know what other traumas he could have encountered on the streets if his parents had not sent for him when they did. The clinical team for this family was distressed to hear that his grandfather had introduced him to adult sexual activities and drugs when he was a mere 5 or 6 years old. It was also disquieting to know that he began performing sexual acts for money and eventually found these activities rewarding enough financially to initiate his own "business"—one that provided him with some financial freedom as well as self-esteem and acceptance, which he had never had previously. Lorenzo bragged to me that he had spent his money on alcohol and marijuana. In spite of this liberal use of substances, he was able to stop drinking and smoking marijuana pretty quickly when he moved to the United States. He confided that he mostly did drugs to alleviate boredom and to fit in with his friends. He also shared that he would rather spend his time playing sports, watching TV, or building puzzles.

Lorenzo noted that his prostitution had started in earnest in the final 3 months before his immigration. As I listened to his story, it almost seemed that his parents' ability to bring him to the United States at this particular time was a miracle of sorts. Had Lorenzo stayed in his home country, the chances were good that his sexual activity would have increased in tandem with the risks. A man had already beaten him up when he was unwilling to turn over for anal intercourse. Instead, Lorenzo kicked him in the groin and ran after being threatened with murder. His friends had told him to lie low, since the man was considered dangerous. When Lorenzo spoke about these experiences, he did so in a distanced fashion.

Structured Assessment Tasks

Drawing Tasks

Lorenzo approached drawing activities with trepidation. He was unable to make a free drawing, and sat in front of the easel and stared. I opted to introduce an activity called the Squiggle Drawing, because it is fun, it is interactive, and it does not require artistic skills. I brought out a piece of paper and two pencils. I told him that his job was to follow my line around the paper, and he did so, laughing a little when I went fast and drew circles and flowing lines. When we finished making tons of little designs, I asked him to look at the page with me and see if he could "see anything that looked like something else." I told him that maybe we could color in things that looked like other things, and he enjoyed pointing to things like "a sun," "a bird," and "a donut," and coloring them in. This art activity was very useful to our relationship building, and it eventually allowed me to proceed and request a self-portrait. Lorenzo made a very light picture of a small figure sitting on a circle. The figure drawing was developmentally regressed, looking as if it was drawn by a much younger child: It had a nondescript head with eyes, nose, and (sad) mouth, and tiny arms with a little circle for hands. The body was another small circle with two small legs coming out of the bottom, and the figure was sitting on a chair. He did not put clothes on the figure and started out with a full torso, erasing over and over until the torso became elongated and phallic-looking. The figure in the chair was placed on top of a large circle. When I looked at it, I asked him to tell me about the picture he had made. He said, "This is me, and I'm sitting on top of the world." (See Figure 10.1.)

My immediate response was that in English, the expression "I'm sitting on top of the world" conveys positive feelings. When I asked Lorenzo what it was like for the person in the drawing to sit on top of the world, he said in a soft voice, "*Triste, no hay puesto para mi en ningún lado*" ("Sad, there is no room for me anywhere"). This metaphor of a child's not fitting anywhere in the world was one we used many times in his subsequent assessment and his therapy, as together we explored how to create a place where he felt that he fitted.

When I asked Lorenzo to draw a family portrait, he said, "I can't."

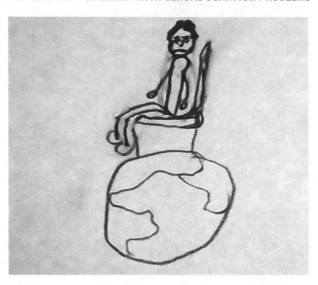

FIGURE 10.1. Lorenzo's drawing: "I'm sitting on top of the world."

When I asked what would happen if he did draw such a picture, he said, "I would have to think about my grandparents, and I don't want to do that." Lorenzo had developed feelings of anger and resentment about his paternal grandparents as he gained the distance he needed to evaluate their treatment of him. Later this anger was redirected toward his parents, and he eventually talked to them directly about why they had left him with people they knew could not take care of him. The family therapy process that followed his individual therapy was deeply painful for both Lorenzo and his parents, but eventually they all had to accept that the choices they had each made in the past had been made without malice and with positive intent, given their circumstances. When Lorenzo accused his father of knowing what his grandparents were capable of doing to Lorenzo, his father sobbed, saying that he had hoped and prayed that his son would be spared. Lorenzo was able to express his sense of being abandoned by his parents and learning to trust no one but himself. He was almost in a rage as he expressed the intense jealousy he felt of his sister, who had lived in the home he should have had, and had basically stolen his life. Lorenzo thought that if Anna Maria had not been born, he would have been brought to the United States much earlier in his life, and his parents would have been more interested in him. It was hard for him to see Anna Maria as innocent in any way;

he perceived her as someone who had robbed him of what was most basic—his parents' love and his right to his childhood. These later family sessions were painful yet necessary, given the varied, intense feelings of all family members.

Sand Therapy

Lorenzo also refused to participate in the play genogram activity, citing the same reasons for his noncompliance. But he was keen on doing sand trays, and his scenarios revealed his deepest longings. His first sand tray was tender and compelling. He put a small table with three chairs and a mother and father rabbit eating with their son, Diego. He then added a heart near the mother figure, and a penguin mother and baby. Last, he added an angel watching over this and titled it "A family having dinner with love." This tray was indicative of the earliest unmet needs he had experienced after his parents left him when he was very young. (See Figure 10.2.)

Lorenzo made limited comments about this sand tray (and others he created during his assessment and treatment), but it was clear that his emotional state changed when he was creating these little scenarios in the sand, using his hands quietly to place things precisely where he wanted them to be. He was very fond of one miniature I had in my collection—a miniature of three angels stuck together. He usually placed these angels in all his sand scenarios. Perhaps they represented a celestial, pure family; perhaps they suggested his carrying his family with him at all times or feeling a non-earthly connection with them. Something had allowed this child to develop glorious resiliency, and when I watched him work, I wondered about a profound sense of spirituality that had perhaps guided and protected him.

Other sand scenarios repeated this initial scene as well as others: villages with children playing outdoors while their parents cooked and watched TV indoors; villages with churches and schools and children who walked together to school; children playing with their dogs, throwing bones that the dogs would return; peaceful, colorful, organized places, probably very different from the places where he had worked.

Later Assessment Impressions

By the time I began to talk to Lorenzo about his sister, his stance on her had softened slightly. He was no longer calling her "fat and ugly"

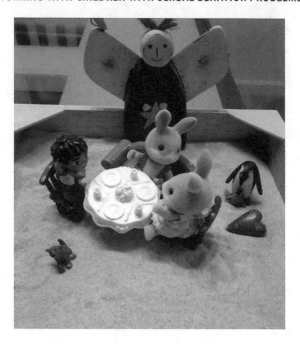

FIGURE 10.2. Lorenzo's sand tray: "A family having dinner with love."

(as he had told the child protective services worker), and he seemed to be starting to understand that she was correct to tell her school counselor after his mother had told her that she would talk to Lorenzo and it wouldn't happen again. (Later, in treatment, Lorenzo had the insight that his mother was capable of great denial. Hilda not only had closed her eyes to Anna Maria when the child had told their mother about Lorenzo, but had closed her eyes to Lorenzo when he had told her that he didn't want to live with his grandparents and begged her to bring him to the United States. Lorenzo said he had cried and pleaded from the time he was 5 years of age, and Hilda had only kept repeating that he would be able to join them soon. This was another understandable resentment that Lorenzo harbored against his mother.)

When we discussed his sexual abuse of his sister, Lorenzo was able to show me what he did, where, and in what sequence the behavior had occurred. He picked up a miniature to represent himself and one to represent his sister (interestingly, they were about the same size). He said the first time he touched her vagina, he had been feeling angry at her all day because she was "annoying." He said that he went into her room at night and asked her to lend him her Game Boy. She whined, refused, and would not tell him where she kept it. He pushed her down into the bed and grabbed her vagina, stating, "You're gonna have to learn to share your things." He said this first time he just grabbed her, but later on, he started making her take off her panties and open her legs, and he touched her and inserted his finger in her. He said he thought she didn't mind what he was doing and didn't seem particularly frightened. After he did this, he would usually feel bad and stay in the room with her, listening to music or playing a game. When I asked him what was going on with his body when he touched her, rubbed her, or put his finger inside her, he said that his penis got "full" and that he liked that feeling. Lorenzo asserted that most of the time when he was touching her initially, he was mad at her, but later he liked the feeling that he got in his penis when he was touching her. He said that he thought about licking her but he was afraid to catch germs from her, and sometimes there was a funny smell that he didn't like. He confided that he had very little experience with girls; in fact, he felt somewhat inadequate and awkward with both girls and women. He was quick to point out that he was not "homosexual," but that his experience had been mostly with men, because they were the ones who sought him out in the night. "I didn't see any women out there paying for sex, just some women selling their bodies." Lorenzo brought up his small size numerous times, and assumed that some people thought he was gay because he was so small. He seemed to be ambivalent about his size: Sometimes he talked about how people were easily fooled into thinking he was weak, and then they were surprised of how well he could take care of himself; at other times, he suggested that in his home country he was not that small, because most people from El Salvador were smaller. His size was certainly noticeable, and it seemed to have many meanings to Lorenzo, depending on the situation.

ASSESSMENT RESULTS

Needless to say, my assessment of Lorenzo was very positive in regard to his ability to be forthcoming about the abuse, his introspection about himself, and the revelations in his work about the unmet nature of his developmental needs. In addition, I felt that Lorenzo was a sensitive and gentle young boy who had a history of complex interpersonal trauma, feelings of abandonment, and a desire to reconnect with his parents and form part of a family that he could love. It was also clear that Lorenzo had experienced inappropriate sexual behaviors, and that in the process he had probably developed some associations between sex and power, or sex and profit. It would be important to uncover how such a young child had managed to perform sexually while compartmentalizing his feelings of fear and confusion. It was also clear that he had not been provided with any parental guidance or any sense of moral values. Finally, his affective life, his dreams, his longings, and his reactions had all been internalized and often kept secret. He had never had the opportunity to feel that he was loved, that he belonged somewhere, and that he would be kept safe and secure. How Lorenzo had done as well as he had was beyond my understanding, other than to suggest that this child had a capacity for transcendence that could have come from a deep spiritual connection—a connection that he could not yet name, but felt.

On the other hand, his sexual abuse of Anna Maria was aggressive, dispassionate, and alarming. Many red flags pointed to Lorenzo's being at high risk of further aggression toward his sister, and the need to engage parental supervision was compelling. I had told Lorenzo that I was concerned about how he spoke about his sister: He seemed to hold her responsible for all his ills, and he objectified her. He seemed surprised that I would be concerned about Anna Maria, given that he perceived her as powerful, but he eventually agreed that he would have to work hard to figure out what to do with his negative feelings toward her. I tried to encourage him to think of Anna Maria and their little brother, Pedro, as very similar—as children who were not responsible for his difficult childhood. However, Lorenzo's feelings were difficult and pervasive, and we agreed that they would be addressed directly in family therapy sessions between him and his parents.

TREATMENT PLAN, GOALS, AND PROCESS

Although Lorenzo seemed receptive to treatment, his treatment needs were overwhelming at times. My first task was to set treatment goals, and I opted to work in individual and group therapy initially to ensure that parental supervision was in place. Individual therapy goals included the following:

1. Obtain Lorenzo's participation in exploring issues related to his sexual abuse of his sister—specifically, his cognitive distortions about the abuse, the feeling states that preceded abuse,

and alternatives to abuse when aggressive or sexual impulses occurred in the future.

2. Discuss Lorenzo's current responses to Anna Maria, and make plans for how to express his thoughts/feelings to others and how to ask for help when needed.

3. Help Lorenzo develop a narrative with cognitive corrections that would provide specific alternatives to sexual abuse.

4. Help him develop alternative, safe, and age-appropriate sexual fantasies.

5. Explore the origins of Lorenzo's sexual knowledge and his early childhood experiences, exploring his cognitive distortions about what is/is not sexual abuse.

6. Explore his feelings and reactions to his grandfather, particularly the grandfather's introducing Lorenzo to explicit sexual activity and substance use.

7. Help Lorenzo understand all household rules related to safety for his sister, himself, and his parents.

In addition to working with him individually, I referred Lorenzo to the Boundary Project (described in Chapter Six), where work began on his sexually aggressive behaviors in a group setting with peers. Lorenzo and his parents attended their own groups, which allowed them to gain knowledge and insight about an array of topics. In addition, when the parents' and children's groups concluded, family members met together to review what they had learned in their own group. Finally, closing rituals in the Boundary Project were playful, relaxing, and provided family members with positive joint experiences.

José and Hilda came to our center twice a week—once to attend the Boundary Project group, and another time to bring Anna Maria to her therapy. The Boundary Project group therapists, myself as Lorenzo's therapist, and Anna Maria's therapist coordinated their work with the home-based worker, Monica. Monica was a tireless advocate for this family, enjoyed being of concrete help to them, and followed all our directives about creating a safe environment for Anna Maria, Lorenzo, and Pedro.

Monica was tasked with ensuring that safety rules were clear, that the parents were supervising and setting limits, and that Lorenzo and Anna Maria were only together when supervised. Lorenzo had learned to avoid Anna Maria on a temporary basis, until he could process his negative feelings toward her. Anna Maria, on the other hand, kept seeking out her brother, not quite understanding why he was always angry with her.

When family therapy began (after Lorenzo and his parents had completed the Boundary Project groups), the goals included the following:

1. Exploration of all family members' deep and intense feelings, which had been left unexpressed for years.
2. Parental explanation for their decision to leave Lorenzo with his paternal grandparents.
3. Improved communication without aggressive language.
4. Parental limit setting about Lorenzo's sexual abuse of his sister, and acknowledgment of both Lorenzo's victimization and his victimizing behaviors and experiences.
5. Systemic realignment to ensure that Lorenzo was welcome in the family, that limits were clear and consistent, that all family members were kept safe, and that family dynamics were open and would not necessitate secrecy.

Eventually Lorenzo began referring to the treatment providers as *"mi gente"* ("my people"), and we gained favor with him. He was particularly fond of the phase of therapy in which I provided Theraplay activities for him and his mother, and eventually for him and his father (Booth & Jernberg, 2010). It was not possible to deliver these attachment-based interventions until other family therapy sessions focused on relational issues were concluded. I believe that the combination of verbal and expressive approaches in our family therapy sessions allowed family members to become more receptive to each other.

SUMMARY AND CONCLUSIONS

Eleven-year-old Lorenzo was referred to our center because he had been sexually abusive to his 6-year-old sister, Anna Maria, for the past 6 months. Because of Lorenzo's age, and because he was not a caretaker to his sister when he abused her, he was allowed to remain in the home; however, the family was referred to ample therapeutic services to ensure the children's safety and to prevent any recurrence of familial sexual abuse.

Lorenzo had been brought to the United States by his family 6 months prior to the referral. Lorenzo had been uprooted from everything familiar, and although he had always wanted to leave El Salvador and join his family, he was ambivalent about the timing because he had recently found a way to establish financial stability. When Lorenzo arrived in the United States, his adjustment was difficult, especially when he discovered that he had to share his parents with two younger siblings who were strangers to him. Lorenzo developed nurturing behaviors toward his 2-year-old brother, Pedro; however, he seemed to take an immediate dislike to his sister, who knew English, seemed happy and well nurtured, and had his parents' devoted attention. Lorenzo developed immediate and intense jealousy of Anna Maria, whom he held responsible for robbing him of his parents' love and a life he'd always wanted. These intense feelings of aggression were merged with sexual acting out, and he had abused his sister without much remorse about the impact of his behavior.

Lorenzo had a history of severe neglect, physical abuse, and sexual abuse. In fact, his grandfather/caretaker had begun prostituting him in order to obtain money for drugs and gambling. Lorenzo's upbringing had been bleak, unsupervised, and unstructured, and he had never been sent to school. He was often hungry, and began pleading with his parents on the phone to bring him to the United States after he turned 5. His confusion about why his parents had left him and why they didn't take him home when he complained about the neglect grew over time. Lorenzo understandably developed ambivalent feelings about his parents, and eventually tried to hold them accountable for "turning a blind eye" to him and his situation and for giving his siblings the life he had not had.

This family came to our clinic in great despair. When following through on the referral from child protective services, they were mostly motivated by fear that Lorenzo would be punished by the criminal justice system—or, even worse, being deported back to his country of origin, El Salvador. The family members' investment in treatment was tenuous at best, and it took great commitment on our part to guide and support them patiently and gently, so they could see us as resources instead of as professionals to be appeased.

Their situation was not unfamiliar to our clinic staff. We often work with immigrant Hispanic families who have sacrificed greatly to obtain a better life for themselves and their children. Often parents come to the United States with high hopes, and they leave their children behind, in the care of trusted extended family. Long periods of time can lapse between the parents' arriving in the United States and their accumulating sufficient resources to send for their children. Many of these young children grow up with very limited contact with their parents, hoping for the day they can be reunited in a new country. On the parents' side, their hopes of financial stability are soon challenged by limited job options (often restricted further by lack of legal residency papers), heavy competition, and high costs of living. Slowly but surely, parents begin to take on multiple jobs, get little sleep, and seem to work as much as possible. In addition, more children are often born in the United States, and these children have a different life from that of their older siblings. When parents finally have the resources to send for their children back home, those children arrive as strangers to their parents, with myriad different experiences. There is an immediate culture shock with different languages and customs, which can leave these newly immigrated children feeling isolated, lonely for their home countries, and overwhelmed by new expectations and demands.

In Lorenzo's case, the family members were very receptive to all the help they were provided. They received specialized victim and victimizer services, which included information on how to respond to both Anna Maria's and Lorenzo's needs. In addition, family therapy was provided in tandem with home-based services designed to ensure the parents' understanding and structuring of a safe environment for their children. A coordinated, structured approach allowed the parents to restore a sense of safety for all their children; it also permitted all family members to make important progress in understanding their prior emotional relationships, build new patterns of communication, and enhance their relationships to each other.

The Boundary Project model for working with children with sexual behavior problems provided a comprehensive, coordinated response in which parents and children participated in their own group sessions, as well as individual and subsequent family therapy sessions. This family made significant changes, and a climate of health and protection was initiated and implemented.

Children with sexual behavior problems must be treated with their families, and their problems must be seen contextually. In this case, the family's cultural practices, immigration, acculturation, and tolerance of abuse had to be explored and understood. In family therapy, José wept when confronted by Lorenzo, who asked pointedly why his father had left him to endure the abuse he knew would be forthcoming. "I didn't know what else to do. I don't know any other kind of life. I thought you would be strong. I thought you would get through as I did." Lorenzo had a difficult time accepting the fact that his father simply believed there was no other course that could be taken, and Lorenzo's forgiveness was slow to come. At the same time, Lorenzo seemed remarkably resilient and resourceful, and responded well to the attention provided to him in individual therapy sessions. In addition, as challenging as it seemed at first, trauma-specific work was undertaken in order to help Lorenzo with his normalization of his abuse. Lorenzo had developed many cognitive distortions about his abuse when he was very young, and overlooked some of the pain he had suffered. In addition, he was slow to recognize his defensive strategies and his ability to compartmentalize his emotions in order to forge ahead. We had many substantive conversations about his prostituting himself, and although I recognized his attempts to regain personal power and control of his life, I also questioned how he had learned to value his sexuality as a bargaining chip for economic freedom. Lorenzo insisted that he viewed sex as a way he could be in control and have power over people; the concepts of "making love" and showing affection and tenderness could not have been farther from his life experience.

Exploring sexuality was not the only arduous topic Lorenzo confronted. Watching Lorenzo try to gain emotional proximity to his parents was heart-wrenching; however, watching them participate in Theraplay activities as well as expressive therapies was deeply satisfying, as these approaches appeared to give them some of the playful, nurturing experiences of childhood and parent–child attachment that both the parents and Lorenzo had missed. These building blocks formed a foundation that allowed for painful confrontations, partial and full forgiveness, and restoration of familial relationships. The sexual behavior problems that brought Lorenzo and his family to treatment were fully responsive to direct and consistent interventions, and the family worked hard to achieve an equilibrium between protection and connection.

As noted earlier, I felt that Lorenzo had a deep spirituality that could account for his resiliency and ability to trust anew. As I grew to know him, and he began to trust the treatment process, he appeared to blossom in response to nurturing attention and earnest support. He expressed himself well; his work in art and sand therapies became profound; and his ability to remain open to new possibilities, was remarkable. Few children have made the impression on me that this child did. Sadly, Hilda could not be moved to break her secret about her daughter's paternity, out of fear of losing her family or incurring her husband's wrath; however, she promised to continue to think about taking that step, given her new understanding that family secrets are usually not helpful and have a way of coming out.

Anna Maria had also shown great resiliency when she approached a school counselor to talk about her brother's abuse, after her mother had told her she would "take care of things" and she did not. Anna Maria was also suffering from ambivalent feelings toward her brother and needed help to understand the effects of the abuse on her. Her parallel treatment process, like Lorenzo's, went well. Eventually conjoint therapy sessions allowed Lorenzo to make an earnest apology for his sexual aggression toward her, and Anna Maria was able to express anger and sadness at being mistreated by him. I can't say that these siblings became close friends, but I do think that they developed a more respectful relationship with each other.

Sexual Contact between Siblings: Normal Sex Play or Problem Behaviors?

The research is clear: Children have a broad range of sexual behaviors, and this range increases gradually as they grow. The research also clearly indicates that a certain amount of normative sexual curiosity or experimentation can occur, especially in families with more than one child (siblings). Because of these findings, we are now in a better position to determine what is or is not normative sexual behavior in children.

All situations involving sexual contact between siblings are unique and must be assessed individually. Rather than using a purely subjective approach, it is important for assessment approaches to be comprehensive and to consider the following important questions:

1. **What is the age difference between the children involved in sexual contact?** Usually, normative sex play can occur between children within a 2-year age range. This means that sex play between children who are no more than 2 years apart is more typical. Large age differences (more than 3 or 4 years) suggest that children are not within the same developmental stages and will usually not have the same level of information or interest in sexual issues.

2. **What is the developmental difference between the children involved?** Children can be similar in chronological age and yet have a significant gap in developmental maturity. Thus assessments

should always consider developmental differences between children (such as the presence of developmental or social delays in one child).

3. **What is the size or status difference between the children involved?** In addition to chronological age and developmental issues, the issues of size and status must be considered. Even when two children are exactly the same age, one child can tower over the other, creating a perception that the larger child has greater power and control. Since sexual abuse usually includes an element of power and control, this issue is relevant. Similarly, a child who is given increased status (for example, a child who is told to take care of another in a parent's absence) also benefits from a perception of unequal power.

4. **Is the type of sexual activity expectable for the children's developmental stage?** Another assessment question involves the type of sexual activity that children initiate. Research states that sexual curiosity, interest, experimentation, and activity gradually increase with age and life experience. For example, it is not expectable that a 4-year-old would know about oral or anal sex, or would initiate this behavior with others. When these behaviors occur out of developmental context, it may suggest that a child has been exposed to explicit sexual information, through either direct experience or viewing of overstimulating materials (such as pornography). Thus it is always important to gauge the sexual activity against the backdrop of what is normative for children of different ages and developmental stages.

5. **Are there elements of coercion, threat, or bribery?** Most common to normative sexual experimentation is the presence of laughter, disinhibition, play, and a sense of doing something a little underhanded. However, in cases of sexual abuse, one child may appear tense, angry, forceful, or manipulative. Sometimes a child obtains compliance from another child by using subtle coercion, withdrawal of friendship, threats to tell others, threats of other negative outcomes, and/or financial or emotional rewards. Sometimes children can be quite forceful or convincing in obtaining other children's compliance, and this may be indicative of non-normative interests that are experienced as compelling.

6. **What are the children's motivations?** As mentioned above, sometimes situations that appear "mutual" may not be. Usually one child initiates behaviors, and this child may have any of a broad range of motivations. For some children, the initiation of sex may be completely based on curiosity and may be fulfilled quickly. For other children, the initiation of sexual activity may emerge from a rich fantasy life and extreme curiosity about sexual matters. Two children can engage in similar acts that can have unique effects on each. It is important, therefore, to gain a clear understanding of the underlying motivations of sexual activities initiated by one child with another.

7. **Is one child isolating another child from others?** When one child initiates sexual activity by isolating another child from others, this could indicate more serious underlying concerns. It is important to be aware of the idiosyncratic nature of motivation and participation in sexual activities in the context of the child's developing sexual maturity, emotional makeup, and other social interactions. For example, sometimes children are angry, have poor emotional regulation, and are generally lacking in social friendships. If these factors are coupled with a focused interest in isolating others for sexual activity, this combination can be a red flag that abusive patterns may be in place.

As mentioned earlier, two children engaged in sexual activity can have completely different experiences of the shared event. It is critical to gauge these unique responses. Some children who are approached for sexual contact may comply out of curiosity, fear, or a need to be seen as "fun" or "cool," or they may simply feel that they have limited options to say no. Whether or not children are outwardly compliant, it is important to look deeper into whether their compliance was experienced as painful, compromising, embarrassing, or otherwise difficult. There are instances when a child appears to be participating, and may even subsequently appear to initiate sexual contact, when in fact the child is asking for attention, for affection, or for the emotional rewards that the activity provides.

Epilogue

It's hard to believe that I (E. G.) first wrote about children with sexual behavior problems in 1992 (with Dr. Toni Cavanagh Johnson). At that time, there was little published research other than Toni's work, although Kee MacFarlane and Carolyn Cunningham were also keeping a focus on this topic with a book originally titled *12 Steps to Healthy Touching* (its second edition is titled simply *Steps to Healthy Touching*; MacFarlane & Cunningham, 2003). If I remember correctly, Kee was the person who coined the phrase "sexually reactive children"; in so doing, she suggested that sexual behavior problems could be reactions to experiences children had endured. I think that this particular phrase reflected sensitivity to young children who were acting out sexually. And sensitivity was needed, because at that time there was a dichotomy between those treatment providers who helped child victims and those who helped victimizers. It is still uncommon to meet mental health professionals who work in both areas, although some of the early polarization has diminished.

When professionals with expertise in working with child victims began to get referrals of children who were victimizing others, responses were varied. Often a child who was exhibiting sexual behavior problems would not be allowed to enter or remain in a program for victims. In the early days of the field, these behaviors in young children truly challenged clinicians and confused their responses. Even today, there is a paucity of specialized services for children with sexual behavior problems.

At this early stage, clinicians struggled to find adequate interventions for young children who showed aggressive sexual acting out toward others. I would love to say that things have improved drastically and that the last 25 years or so have made a remarkable difference. But it really doesn't feel that way. This topic still feels confusing and challenging, and it remains very misunderstood. Either parents are still ignoring behaviors in their children that make them uncomfortable, or they are rushing for help prematurely, before making reasonable efforts to understand and correct the behaviors themselves.

The reality is that the area of sexuality in general, and childhood sexuality specifically, continues to be clouded in secrecy and misinformation. Even though more and more information has become available to parents on childhood sexuality (see, e.g., the list of books for parents in the Resources section following this Epilogue), parents don't seem to achieve sufficient clarity or confidence to deal with their children's normative sexual development, much less the sexual behavior problems that can arise.

Likewise, many more professional books on this topic have become available over the last two decades, as has research that points to promising interventions. The Association for the Treatment of Sexual Abusers (ATSA) commissioned a Task Force to summarize available information on children and adolescents with sexual behavior problems, and the resulting report is widely cited in this book (Chaffin et al., 2006). This report is enlightening and truly appears to be the definitive treatise on the subject to date.

My (E.G.) clinical interest in sexual behavior problems in children has continued throughout my now 40-year professional career in child abuse prevention and treatment. I'm proud of my life's work and my ongoing efforts to learn more ways of helping the children and families I treat. My job has been very rewarding overall, and over time, some of the challenges that felt overwhelming now feel manageable as my experiences provide more direction. In addition, most clinicians learn through equal amounts of formal education, continuing education, and on-the-job learning. This has certainly been true for me! I have had hundreds of opportunities to meet with families in crisis—parents who have recently discovered that their children have hurt someone; parents who find themselves torn between their desire to protect one of their children, and to punish and chastise another. In my experience, no pain seems greater than the pain of sibling incest for parents who have to negotiate intense feelings toward two (or more) children whom they love. Feelings of despair, anger, betrayal, fear, guilt, and shame seem pervasive in my work with the families of children with sexual behavior problems.

At this time in my career, I feel that my grasp of the issues involved in treatment is fairly secure. Although a completely structured blueprint for how to proceed in these cases is not yet available, I believe that there is a course of action that usually serves our families well. I feel able to reassure parents sincerely, because I believe that things can improve. I am able to share optimism because I have seen incredible gains when families are in treatment. I am no longer frightened or reluctant to work with children who appear ambivalent or hesitant, withdrawn or enraged, because I am confident that with time their hard exteriors will soften. I am able to trust that the process of therapy can and does help, and I feel confident to offer services that others before me have also found useful to families.

But it is clearly a different world from the one I knew as a child, and my grandchildren will face different challenges and be given different opportunities than I could have ever fathomed. Some of the changes are glorious and make life so much more exciting; other changes are daunting and loom over us with grave implications.

As we have described in detail in Chapter Three, the mass media appear to be sexualizing younger and younger children, and young children are clearly the targets of massive sex-based marketing schemes. Sexuality is used to sell products, and children have more explicit information at their fingertips than ever before. When I was a child, my brother and I looked forward to *National Geographic* to catch a glimpse of a nude body. These days, the sheer amount of explicit material available from various sources, and the provocative nature of much of it, is simply astonishing. Young children have many more ways of accessing information about sexuality than ever before. Some of this material is "live," not just print—and it provides an array of sexual activity that includes young children and adults, as well as overt acts of violence.

I don't think any of us could have imagined this onslaught of explicit sexual information or the easy access that children would have to it. I don't mean to suggest that there is a linear cause-and-effect relationship between looking at sexual print or video and acting out—but I do think that many young children can become fascinated by sexual activity, may not understand their physical and emotional reactions to what they see, and may not have the adult guidance that would enable them to properly assess what they are looking at. And yes, some children may begin to experiment in ways they would not have done if they had not been exposed to overstimulating material. Our practices are full of these young children.

During the writing of this book, the tragedy of Newtown, Connecticut, occurred. The Newtown massacre left us all breathless, shocked, profoundly saddened, and frightened. These tragedies have intruded into our insulated sense of safety and caused deep introspection. There was a great deal of dispassionate discussion following the shooting deaths of 27 people in Sandy Hook Elementary School, and there is always the temptation to try to find a single explanation for the unthinkable. But there is never just one explanation for things we find challenging to comprehend, and Newtown is just one more example of this. So even as this book has attempted to find plausible explanations for why children become inexplicably sexually aggressive toward others or develop other sexual behavior problems, we always need to look at the bigger picture, and consider all the possible variables that can contribute to problems of any type.

Even the challenges of living in this new world do not negate the fact that it is also an exciting time to be a practicing mental health professional. The available information keeps growing, and professionals are increasingly invested in learning more and providing more effective treatment outcomes. The growing numbers of practice- and evidence-informed programs contribute to inform the development of our therapeutic directions and specific goals. And while theories, techniques, and approaches abound, I prioritize something that cannot be taught: a willingness to engage emotionally with clients; to anchor clients in a stable and predictable relationship; and to trust in children's (and their parents') ability to overcome challenges, strive for something better, and achieve positive gains.

Resources

BIBLIOGRAPHY FOR PARENTS*

Haffner, D. W. (1999). *From diapers to dating: A parent's guide to raising sexually healthy children.* New York: Newmarket Press.—This
book is filled with practical advice and guidelines to help parents
and other caregivers feel more comfortable talking to children and
early adolescents about sexual issues. Incorporating value exercises,
it encourages parents to examine their own sexual values so that
they can share these messages with their children.

Haffner, D. W. (2008). *Beyond the big talk: A parent's guide to raising
sexually healthy teens.* New York: Newmarket Press.—This book
helps parents and caregivers address sexual issues with their adolescents. It provides specific information for each age group: middle school (grades 7–8), early high school (grades 9–10), late high
school (grades 11–12), and beyond (ages 19 and up).

Haffner, D. W. (2008). *What every 21st-century parent needs to know:
Facing today's challenges with wisdom and heart.* New York: Newmarket Press.—This book was written to debunk the myths, vali-
date the concerns, and advise parents on how to keep their children
safe and healthy in a world so different from the one in which they
grew up. The author addresses the good and bad news about 21st-
century parents' concerns, including stress, self-esteem, drinking,
achievement, drugs, Internet safety, cell phones, Facebook, depression, sports, nutrition, bullying, faith, abstinence, and sex.

---

* Provided by the Sexuality Information and Education Council of the United
States.

Johnson, T. C. (1999). *Understanding your child's sexual behavior: What's natural and healthy.* Oakland, CA: New Harbinger.— This book addresses healthy and unhealthy sexual behaviors of children and adolescents from birth to 12 years of age. It provides parents/caregivers and professionals with information to help identify, understand, and respond appropriately to these behaviors.

Levkoff, L. (2007). *Third base ain't what it used to be: What your kids are learning about sex today—and how to teach them to become sexually healthy adults.* New York: New American Library.—In a straightforward style, this book offers advice for parents and caregivers who are struggling to answer their kids' questions about sexuality or just trying to bring up the topic in the first place. The author offers guidance on discussing everything from gender issues, body image, and sexual orientation to AIDS and abortion.

Richardson, J., & Schuster, M. A. (2003). *Everything you never wanted your kids to know about sex (but were afraid they'd ask): The secrets to surviving your child's sexual development from birth to the teens.* New York: Crown.—This book is written for parents and other caregivers of children of all ages; it covers childhood sexual development in stages, introducing issues for each and how to discuss them. The authors accommodate variations in values, from "teen sex is fine" to "save it for marriage," and support their advice with scholarly research and stories from real parents about what worked—and didn't—with their kids.

Roffman, D. M. (2002). *But how'd I get in there in the first place?: Talking to your young child about sex.* Cambridge, MA: Perseus.— This book, written for parents and caregivers of children 3–6 years old, is intended to help parents begin talking about sexuality, conception, and birth. The author believes that the key to talking with children about sexuality is knowing that their questions fall into three easily recognizable categories.

Roffman, D. M. (2001). *Sex and sensibility: The thinking parent's guide to talking sense about sex.* Cambridge, MA: Perseus.—This book is designed to help parents and other caregivers open the lines of communication about sexuality with their children, interpret and respond to virtually any question a child might pose, and deal with any situation that may arise.

Schwartz, P., & Cappello, D. (2000). *Ten talks parents must have with their children about sex and character.* New York: Hyperion.—This book was written for parents and caregivers of children in grades 4–12 to help them talk about sexuality and building character.

Topics include safety, character, peer pressure, ethics, the Internet, and the media.

Schwier, K. M., & Hingsburger, D. (2000). *Sexuality: Your sons and daughters with intellectual disabilities*. Baltimore: Brookes.—This book provides information, advice, and practical strategies to parents and other caregivers on interacting with their children—no matter what their age or ability—in a way that increases their self-esteem, encourages appropriate behavior, empowers them to recognize and respond to abuse, and enables them to develop lifelong relationships.

PROFESSIONAL ORGANIZATIONS

American Art Therapy Association (AATA)
4875 Eisenhower Avenue, Suite 240
Alexandria, VA 22304
888-290-0878
www.arttherapy.org

Association for Play Therapy (APT)
3198 Willow Avenue, Suite 110
Clovis, CA 93612-4716
559-294-2128
www.a4pt.org

Sandplay Therapists of America (STA)
P.O. Box 4847
Walnut Creek, CA 94596
925-820-2109
www.sandplay.org

RECOMMENDED TEXTS FOR CLINICIANS

American Academy of Pediatrics. (2005). *Sexual behaviors in children*. Elk Grove Village, IL: Author.

Araji, S. K. (1997). *Sexually aggressive children: Coming to understand them*. Thousand Oaks, CA: Sage.

Carpentier, M. Y., Silovsky, J. F., & Chaffin, M. (2006). Randomized trial of treatment for children with sexual behavior problems: Ten-year follow-up. *Journal of Consulting and Clinical Psychology, 74*(3), 482–488.

Chaffin, M., Berliner, L., Block, R., Johnson, T. C., Friedrich, W., Louis, D. G., et al. (2006). *Report of the Task Force on Children with Sexual Behavior Problems*. Beaverton, OR: Association for the Treatment of Sexual Abusers. Retrieved from *www.atsa.com/atsa-csb-task-force-report*.

Friedrich, W. N. (2002). *Psychological assessment of sexually abused children and their families*. Thousand Oaks, CA: Sage.

Friedrich, W. N. (2007). *Children with sexual behavior problems: Family-based, attachment-focused therapy*. New York: Norton.

Friedrich, W. N., Fisher, J., Broughton, D., Houston, M., & Shafran, C. R. (1998). Normative sexual behavior in children: A contemporary sample. *Pediatrics, 101*(4), E9.

Gil, E., & Johnson, T. C. (1993). *Sexualized children: Assessment and treatment of sexualized children and children who molest*. Royal Oak, MI: Self-Esteem Shop.

Hagan, J. F., Shaw, J. S., & Duncan, P. (Eds.). (2008). Theme 8: Promoting healthy sexual development and sexuality. In *Bright futures: Guidelines for health supervision of infants, children, and adolescents* (3rd ed., pp. 169–176). Elk Grove Village, IL: American Academy of Pediatrics.

Pithers, W. D., Gray, A., Busconi, A., & Houchens, P. (1998). Children with sexual behavior problems: Identification of five distinct child types and related treatment considerations. *Child Maltreatment, 3*(4), 384–406.

Silvosky, J. F., & Niec, L. (2002). Characteristics of young children with sexual behavior problems: A pilot study. *Child Maltreatment, 7*, 187–197.

References

Abramson, E., & Valene, P. (1991). Media use, dietary restraint, bulimia, and attitudes towards obesity: A preliminary study. *British Review of Bulimia and Anorexia Nervosa, 5,* 73–76.

Achenbach, T. M., & Rescorla, L. A. (2000). *Manual for the ASEBA Preschool Forms & Profiles.* Burlington: University of Vermont, Research Center for Children, Youth & Families.

Achenbach, T. M., & Rescorla, L. A. (2001). *Manual for the ASEBA School-Age Forms & Profiles.* Burlington: University of Vermont, Research Center for Children, Youth & Families.

Ainsworth, M. D. S., Blehar, M. C., Waters, E., & Wall, S. (1978). *Patterns of attachment: A psychological study of the strange situation.* Hillsdale, NJ: Erlbaum.

American Academy of Child and Adolescent Psychiatry. (1997). Practice parameters for the forensic evaluation of children and adolescents who may have been physically or sexually abused. *Journal of the American Academy of Child and Adolescent Psychiatry, 36,* 423–442.

American Academy of Pediatrics. (2005). *Sexual behaviors in children.* Elk Grove Village, IL: Author.

American Psychological Association (APA) Task Force on the Sexualization of Girls. (2007, February 19). Executive summary. Retrieved from *www.apa. org/pi/women/programs/girls/report.*

Araji, S. K. (1997). *Sexually aggressive children: Coming to understand them.* Thousand Oaks, CA: Sage.

Bakermans-Kranenburg, M. J., van IJzendoorn, M. H., & Juffer, F. (2003). Less is more: Meta-analyses of sensitivity and attachment interventions in early childhood. *Psychological Bulletin, 129*(2), 195–215.

Barkley, R. A., & Benton, C. M. (2013). *Your defiant child: Eight steps to better behavior* (2nd ed.). New York: Guilford Press.

Blaustein, M. E., & Kinniburgh, K. M. (2010). *Treating traumatic stress in children and adolescents: How to foster resilience through attachment, self-regulation, and competency.* New York: Guilford Press.

Bonner, B. L., & Fahey, W. E. (1998). Children with aggressive sexual behavior. In A. S. Bellack & M. Hersen (Series Eds.) & N. N. Singh & A .S. W. Winton (Vol. Eds.), *Comprehensive clinical psychology: Vol. 9. Clinical psychology: Special populations* (pp. 453–466). Oxford, UK: Elsevier.

Bonner, B. L., Walker, C. E., & Berliner, L. (1999). *Children with sexual behavior problems: Assessment and treatment* (Final Report, Grant No. 90-CA-1469). Washington, DC: U.S. Department of Health and Human Services, National Clearinghouse on Child Abuse and Neglect.

Booth, P. B., & Jernberg, A. M. (2010). *Theraplay: Helping parents and children build better relationships through attachment-based play* (3rd ed.). San Francisco: Jossey-Bass.

Bowlby, J. (1988). On knowing what you are not supposed to know and feeling what you are not supposed to feel. In J. Bowlby (Ed.), *A secure base: Parent–child attachments and healthy human development* (pp. 99–118). New York: Basic Books.

Brestan, E. V., & Eyberg, S. M. (1998). Effective psychosocial treatments for children and adolescents with disruptive behavior disorders: 29 years, 82 studies, and 5272 kids. *Journal of Clinical Child Psychology, 27,* 179–188.

Briere, J. (1996). *Trauma Symptom Checklist for Children: Professional manual.* Lutz, FL: Psychological Assessment Resources.

Briere, J. (2005). *Trauma Symptom Checklist for Young Children: Professional manual.* Lutz, FL: Psychological Assessment Resources.

Brotto, L., Heiman, J., & Tolman, D. (2009). Narratives of desire in mid-age women with and without arousal difficulties. *Journal of Sex Research, 46*(5), 387–398.

Calvert, S. (2008). Children as consumers: Advertising and marketing. *The Future of Children, 18*(1), 205–234.

Carey, L. (1999). *Sandplay therapy with children and families.* Northvale, NJ: Aronson.

Chaffin, M., Berliner, L., Block, R., Johnson, T. C., Friedrich, W., Louis, D. G., et al. (2006). *Report of the Task Force on Children with Sexual Behavior Problems.* Beaverton, OR: Association for the Treatment of Sexual Abusers. Retrieved from *www.atsa.com/atsa-csb-task-force-report.*

Chaffin, M., Letourneau, E., & Silovsky, J. F. (2002). Adults, adolescents, and children who sexually abuse children: A developmental perspective. In J. E. B. Myers, L. Berliner, J. Briere, C. Jenny, T. Hendrix, & T. E. Reid (Eds.), *The APSAC handbook on child maltreatment* (2nd ed., pp. 205–232). Thousand Oaks, CA: Sage.

Cohen, J. A., & Mannarino, A. P. (1993). A treatment model for sexually abused preschoolers. *Journal of Interpersonal Violence, 8*(1), 115–131.

Cohen, J. A., & Mannarino, A. P. (1996). Factors that mediate treatment outcome in sexually abused preschool children: Initial findings. *Journal of the American Academy of Child and Adolescent Psychiatry, 35*(10), 1402–1410.

Cohen, J. A., & Mannarino, A. P. (1997). The Weekly Behavior Report: A parent-report instrument for sexually abused preschoolers. *Child Maltreatment, 1,* 353–360.

Cohen, J. A., Mannarino, A. P., & Deblinger, E. (2006). *Treating trauma and traumatic grief in children and adolescents*. New York: Guilford Press.

Cook, J. (2007). *Personal space camp*. Chattanooga, TN: National Center for Youth Issues.

Deblinger, E., & Heflin, A. H. (1996). *Treating sexually abused children and their nonoffending parents*. Thousand Oaks, CA: Sage.

Deblinger, E., Stauffer, L. B., & Steer, R.A. (2001). Comparative efficacies of supportive and cognitive behavioral group therapies for young children who have been sexually abused and their nonoffending mothers. *Child Maltreatment, 6,* 332–343.

Drewes, A. A., & Cavett, A. M. (2012). Play applications and skills components. In J. A. Cohen, A. P. Mannarino, & E. Deblinger (Eds.), *Trauma-focused CBT for children and adolescents: Treatment applications* (pp. 105–123). New York: Guilford Press.

Durham, M. G. (2008). *The Lolita effect: The media sexualization of young girls and what we can do about it*. New York: The Overlook Press.

Durkin, S. J., & Paxton, S. J. (2002). Predictors of vulnerability to reduced body image satisfaction and psychological wellbeing in response to exposure to idealized female body images in adolescent girls. *Journal of Psychosomatic Research, 53,* 995–1005.

Eder, D. (with Evans, C. C., & Parker, S.). (1995). *School talk: Gender and adolescent culture*. New Brunswick, NJ: Rutgers University Press.

Farmer, E., & Pollock, S. (1998). *Sexually abused and abusing children in substitute care*. New York: Wiley.

Fredrickson, B. L., & Roberts, T. A. (1997). Objectification theory: Toward understanding women's lived experience and mental health risks. *Psychology of Women Quarterly, 21,* 173–206.

Fredrickson, B. L., Roberts, T. A., Noll, S. M., Quinn, D. M., & Twenge, J. M. (1998). That swimsuit becomes you: Sex differences in self-objectification, restrained eating, and math performance. *Journal of Personality and Social Psychology, 75,* 269–284.

Friedrich, W. N. (1997). *Child Sexual Behavior Inventory: Professional manual*. Odessa, FL: Psychological Assessment Resources.

Friedrich, W. N. (2007). *Children with sexual behavior problems: Family-based, attachment-focused therapy*. New York: Norton.

Friedrich, W. N., Davies, W., Feher, E., & Wright, J. (2003). Sexual behavior problems in preteen children: Developmental, ecological, and behavioral correlates. *Annals of the New York Academy of Sciences, 989,* 95–104.

Friedrich, W. N., Fisher, J., Broughton, D., Houston, M., & Shafran, C. R. (1998). Normative sexual behavior in children: A contemporary sample. *Pediatrics, 101*(4), E9.

Friedrich, W. N., Fisher, J. L., Dittner, C., Acton, R., Berliner, L., Butler, J., et al. (2001). Child Sexual Behavior Inventory: Normative, psychiatric, and sexual abuse comparisons. *Child Maltreatment, 6,* 37–49.

Friedrich, W. N., Grambsch, P., Broughton, D., Kuiper, J., & Beilke, R. L. (1991). Normative sexual behavior in children. *Pediatrics, 88,* 456–464.

Friedrich, W. N., Luecke, W. M., Beilke, R. L., & Place, V. (1992). Psychotherapy outcome of sexually abused boys. *Journal of Interpersonal Violence, 7,* 396–409.

Gapinski, K. D., Brownell, K. D., & LaFrance, M. (2003). Body objectification and "fat talk": Effects on emotion, motivation, and cognitive performance. *Sex Roles, 48,* 377–388.

Gerard, A. B. (1994). *Parent–Child Relationship Inventory manual.* Los Angeles: Western Psychological Services.

Gerbner, G. (1994). Reclaiming our cultural mythology: Television's global marketing strategy creates a damaging and alienated window on the world. *The Ecology of Justice, No. 38.* Retrieved from *www.context.org/iclib/ic38/gerbner.*

Gil, E. (1993). Age-appropriate sex play versus problematic sexual behaviors. In E. Gil & T. C. Johnson, *Sexualized children: Assessment and treatment of sexualized children and children who molest* (pp. 21–40). Royal Oak, MI: Self-Esteem Shop.

Gil, E. (2003a). Family play therapy: "The bear with short nails." In C. E. Schaefer (Ed.), *Foundations of play therapy* (pp. 192–218). Hoboken, NJ: Wiley.

Gil, E. (2003b). Play genograms. In C. F. Sori, L. L. Hecker, & Associates (Eds.), *The therapist's notebook for children and adolescents: Homework, handouts, and activities for use in psychotherapy* (pp. 49–56). Binghamton, NY: Haworth Clinical Practice Press.

Gil, E. (2010a). *The extended play-based developmental assessment manual.* Royal Oak, MI: Self-Esteem Shop.

Gil, E., (Ed.). (2010b). *Working with children to heal interpersonal trauma: The power of play.* New York: Guilford Press.

Gil, E. (2012). Trauma-focused integrated play therapy. In P. Goodyear-Brown (Ed.), *Handbook of child sexual abuse: Identification, assessment, and treatment* (pp. 251–278). Hoboken, NJ: Wiley.

Gil, E., & Johnson, T. C. (1993). *Sexualized children: Assessment and treatment of sexualized children and children who molest.* Royal Oak, MI: Self-Esteem Shop.

Gil, E., & Shaw, J. (2010). *A book for kids about private parts, touching, touching problems, and other stuff.* Royal Oak, MI: Self-Esteem Shop.

Giordano, M., Landreth, G., & Jones, L. (2005). *Practical handbook for building the play therapy relationship.* Lanham, MD: Aronson.

Gitlin-Weiner, K., Sandgrund, A., & Schaefer, C. E. (Eds.). (2000). *Play diagnosis and assessment* (2nd ed.). New York: Wiley.

Gottman, J. (1997). *Raising an emotionally intelligent child: The heart of parenting.* New York: Fireside/Simon & Schuster.

Grant, R. K., & Lundeberg, L. H. (2009). *Interventions for children with sexual behavior problems: Research, theory, and treatment.* Kingston, NJ: Civic Research Institute.

Greenspan, S. I. (2002). *The secure child: Helping our children feel safe and confident in a changing world.* Cambridge, MA: Da Capo Press.

Greco, L. A., & Hayes, S. C. (2008). *Acceptance and mindfulness treatments for children and adolescents: A practitioner's guide.* Oakland, CA: New Harbinger.

Hagan, J. F., Shaw, J. S., & Duncan, P. M. (Eds.). (2008). *Bright futures:*

Guidelines for health supervision of infants, children, and adolescents (3rd ed.). Elk Grove Village, IL: American Academy of Pediatrics.

Hall, D., Mathews, F., Pearce, J., Sarlo-McGarvey, N., & Gavin, D. (1996). *The development of sexual behavior problems.* South Pasadena, CA: Authors.

Harrison, K. (2000). The body electric: Thin-ideal media and eating disorders in adolescents. *Journal of Communication, 50*(3), 119–143.

Hawn, G. (with Holden, W.). (2011). *10 mindful minutes: Giving our children and ourselves the social and emotional skills to reduce stress and anxiety for healthier, happier lives.* New York: Perigee/Penguin Group.

Hebl, M. R., King, E. G., & Lin, J. (2004). The swimsuit becomes us all: Ethnicity, gender, and vulnerability to self-objectification. *Personality and Social Psychology Bulletin, 30*, 1322–1331.

Hembree-Kigin, T. L., & McNeil, C. (1995). *Parent–child interaction therapy.* New York: Plenum Press.

Herman, J. L. (1992). *Trauma and recovery.* New York: Basic Books.

Hofschire, L., & Greenberg, B. (2002). Media's impact on adolescents' body dissatisfaction. In J. Brown, J. Steele, & K. Walsh-Childers (Eds.), *Sexual teens, sexual media: Investigating media's influence on adolescent sexuality* (pp. 125–149). Mahwah, NJ: Erlbaum.

Homeyer, L., & Sweeney, D. (2011). *Sandtray therapy: A practical manual* (2nd ed.). Royal Oak, MI: Self-Esteem Shop.

Impett, E. A., Schooler, D., & Tolman, D. L. (2006). To be seen and not heard: Femininity ideology and adolescent girls' sexual health. *Archives of Sexual Behavior, 21*, 628–646.

Jaffe, A. V., & Gardner, L. (2006). *My book full of feelings: An interactive workbook for parents, professionals, and children.* Shawnee Mission, KS: Autism Asperger Publishing.

Kaeser, F. (2011). *What your child needs to know about sex (and when): A straight talking guide for parents.* New York: Random House.

Kaeser, F. (2011, Sept 23). The super-sexualization of children: Time to take notice. *Psychology Today. www.psychologytoday.com/blog/what-your-child-needs-know-about-sex-and-when/201109/the-super-sexualization-children-time-take.*

Karst, P. (2000). *The invisible string.* Camarillo, CA: DeVorss.

Kaufman, S. H., & Burns, R. C. (1972). *Actions, styles, and symbols in kinetic family drawings: An interpretative manual.* New York: Brunner/Mazel.

Kellogg, N. D., & Committee on Child Abuse and Neglect. (2009). Clinical report: The evaluation of sexual behaviors in children. *Pediatrics, 124*, 992–998.

Kendall-Tackett, K., Williams, L. M., & Finkelhor, D. (1993). Impact of sexual abuse on children: A review and synthesis of recent empirical studies. *Psychological Bulletin, 113*, 164–180.

Kunkel, D., Eyal, K., Finnerty, K., Biely, E., & Donnerstein, E. (2005). *Sex on TV 4.* Menlo Park, CA: Kaiser Family Foundation. Retrieved March 25, 2008, from *www.kff.org/entmedia/upload/Sex-on-TV-4-Full-Report.pdf.*

Labovitz Boik, B., & Goodwin, E. A. (2000). *Sandplay therapy: A step-by-step manual for psychotherapists of diverse orientations.* New York: Norton.

Lamb, S. (2006). *Sex, therapy, and kids: Addressing their concerns through talking and play*. New York: Norton.

Lamb-Shapiro, J. (2000). *The hyena who lost her laugh: A story about changing your negative thinking*. Woodbury, NY: Childswork/Childsplay.

Landreth, G. L. (2012). *Play therapy: The art of the relationship* (3rd ed.). New York: Routledge.

Landreth, G. L., & Bratton, S. C. (2006). *Child parent relationship therapy (CPRT): A 10-session filial therapy model*. New York: Routledge.

Landreth, G. L., Sweeney, D. S., Homeyer, L. E., Ray, D. C., & Glover, G. J. (2005). *Play therapy interventions with children's problems: Case studies with DSM-IV-TR diagnoses* (2nd ed.). Lanham, MD: Aronson.

Langstrom, N., Grann, M., & Lichtenstein, P. (2002). Genetic and environmental influences on problematic masturbatory behavior in children: A study of same-sex twins. *Archives of Sexual Behavior, 31*, 343–350.

Levin, D. E., & Kilbourne, J. (2008). *So sexy so soon: The new sexualized childhood, and what parents can do to protect their kids*. New York: Ballantine Books.

Lieberman, A. F., & Van Horn, P. (2008). *Psychotherapy with infants and young children: Repairing the effects of stress and trauma on early attachment*. New York: Guilford Press.

MacFarlane, K., & Cunningham, C. (2003). *Steps to healthy touching: Activities to help kids understand and control their problems with touching* (2nd ed.). Amsterdam: KidsRights.

Malchiodi, C. (1998). *Understanding children's drawings*. New York: Guilford Press.

McGoldrick, M., Gerson, R., & Petry, S. (2008). *Genograms: Assessment and intervention* (3rd ed.). New York: Norton.

McKinley, N. M., & Hyde, J. S. (1996). The Objectified Body Consciousness Scale. *Psychology of Women Quarterly, 20*, 181–215.

Merrick, M., Litrownik, A., Everson, M., & Cox, C. (2008). Beyond sexual abuse: The impact of other maltreatment experiences on sexualized behaviors. *Child Maltreatment, 13*, 122–132.

Mills, J. S., Polivy, J., Herman, P., & Tiggemann, M. (2002). Effects of exposure to thin media images: Evidence of self-enhancement among restrained eaters. *Personality and Social Psychology Bulletin, 28*(12), 1687–1699.

Mitchell, R. R., & Friedman, S. H. (1994). *Sandplay: Past, present, and future*. New York: Routledge.

Narelle, B. (2011). *Thinkafeeladoo: JoJo's not so great day*. Available from *www.lulu.com/us/en/shop*.

Nichter, M. (2000). *Fat talk: What girls and their parents say about dieting*. Cambridge, MA: Harvard University Press.

O'Donohue, W., Gold, S. R., & McKay, J. S. (1997). Children as sexual objects: Historical and gender trends in magazines. *Sexual Abuse: Journal of Research and Treatment, 9*, 291–301.

Patterson, G. R., Reid, J. B., & Eddy, J. M. (2002). A brief history of the Oregon model. In J. B. Reid, G. R. Patterson, & J. Snyder (Eds.), *Antisocial* behavior in children and adolescents: A developmental analysis and model for intervention (pp. 3–20). Washington, DC: American Psychological Association.

Pennsylvania Coalition Against Rape. (n.d.). Three Kinds of Touches curriculum. Enola: Author.

Perry, B. (2009). Examining child maltreatment through a neurodevelopmental lens: Clinical applications of the neurosequential model of therapeutics. Journal of Loss and Trauma, 14, 240–255.

Peterson, L. W., & Hardin, M. E. (1997). Children in distress: A guide for screening children's art. New York: Norton.

Pithers, W. D., & Gray, A. S. (1993). Pre-adolescent sexual abuse research project: Research grantees status report. Washington, DC: National Center on Child Abuse and Neglect.

Pithers, W. D., Gray, A., Busconi, A., & Houchens, P. (1998). Children with sexual behavior problems: Identification of five distinct child types and related treatment considerations. Child Maltreatment, 3(4), 384–406.

Rideout, V. J., Vandewater, E. A., & Wartella, E. A. (2003). Zero to six: Electronic media in the lives of infants, toddlers and preschoolers. Menlo Park, CA: Kaiser Family Foundation.

Rubin, J. A. (2005). Child art therapy (25th anniversary ed.). Hoboken, NJ: Wiley.

Sanders, M. R., Cann, W., & Markie-Dadds, C. (2003). The Triple P-Positive Parenting Programme: A universal population-level approach to the prevention of child abuse. Child Abuse Review, 12, 155–171.

Schaefer, C. E. (Ed.). (1993). The therapeutic powers of play. Northvale, NJ: Aronson.

Schaefer, C. E. (Ed.). (2003). Foundations of play therapy. Hoboken, NJ: Wiley.

Siegel, D. J., & Payne Bryson, T. (2011). The whole-brain child: 12 revolutionary strategies to nurture your child's developing mind. New York: Delacorte.

Silovsky, J. F., & Bonner, B. L. (2003a). Children with sexual behavior problems: Common misconceptions vs. current findings (Fact Sheet No. 2). Oklahoma City, OK: National Center on Sexual Behavior of Youth.

Silovsky, J. F., & Bonner, B. L. (2003b). Sexual behavior problems. In T. H. Ollendick & C. S. Schroeder (Eds.), Encyclopedia of clinical child and pediatric psychology (pp. 589–591). New York: Kluwer Academic/Plenum.

Silovsky, J. F., & Bonner, B. L. (2004). Sexual development and sexual behavior problems in children ages 2–12 (Fact Sheet No. 4). Oklahoma City, OK: National Center on Sexual Behavior of Youth.

Silovsky, J. F., & Niec, L. (2002). Characteristics of young children with sexual behavior problems: A pilot study. Child Maltreatment, 7, 187–197.

Silovsky, J. F., Niec, L., Bard, D., & Hecht, D. (2007). Treatment for preschool children with interpersonal sexual behavior problems: Pilot study. Journal of Clinical Child and Adolescent Psychology, 36, 378–391.

Silovsky, J. F., Swisher, L. M., Widdifield, J., Jr., & Burris, L. (2012). Clinical considerations when children have problematic sexual behavior. In P.

Goodyear-Brown (Ed.), *Handbook of child sexual abuse: Identification, assessment, and treatment* (pp. 401–428). Hoboken, NJ: Wiley.

Slater, A., & Tiggemann, M. (2002). A test of objectification theory in adolescent girls. *Sex Roles, 46,* 343–349.

Sobol, B., & Schneider, K. (1998). Art as an adjunctive therapy in the treatment of children who dissociate. In J. L. Silberg (Ed.), *The dissociative child: Diagnosis, treatment and management* (pp. 191–218). Luthersville, MD: Sidran Press.

Stallard, P. (2002). *Think good—feel good: A cognitive behaviour therapy workbook for children and young people.* Chichester, UK: Wiley.

Stauffer, L. B., & Deblinger, E. (1996). Cognitive behavioral groups for nonoffending mothers and their young sexually abused children: A preliminary treatment outcome study. *Child Maltreatment, 1,* 65–76.

Stice, E., Schupak-Neuberg, E., Shaw, H. E., & Stein, R. I. (1994). Relation of media exposure to eating disorder symptomatology: An examination of mediating mechanisms. *Journal of Abnormal Psychology, 103*(4), 836–840.

Thomsen, S. R., Weber, M. M., & Brown, L. B. (2002). The relationship between reading beauty and fashion magazines and the use of pathogenic dieting methods among adolescent females. *Adolescence, 37,* 1–18.

Turner, B. A. (2005). *The handbook of sandplay therapy.* Cloverdale, CA: Temenos Press.

Ward, L. M. (2002). Does television exposure affect emerging adults' attitudes and assumptions about sexual relationships?: Correlational and experimental confirmation. *Journal of Youth and Adolescence, 31,* 1–15.

Ward, L. M. (2004). Wading through the stereotypes: Positive and negative associations between media use and black adolescents' conceptions of self. *Developmental Psychology, 40,* 284–294.

Ward, L. M., & Rivadeneyra, R. (1999). Contributions of entertainment television to adolescents' sexual attitudes and expectations: The role of viewing amount versus viewer involvement. *Journal of Sex Research, 36,* 237–249.

Webster-Stratton, C. (2006). *The incredible years: A trouble-shooting guide for parents of children aged 2–8 years.* Seattle, WA: Incredible Years.

White, S., Halpin, B. M., Strom, G. A., & Santilli, G. (1988). Behavioral comparisons of young sexually abused, neglected, and nonreferred children. *Journal of Clinical Child Psychology, 17,* 53–61.

Wilcox, B. L., Kunkel, D., Cantor, J., Dowrick, P., Linn, S., & Palmer, E. (2004, February 20). *Report of the APA Task Force on Advertising and Children.* Washington, DC: American Psychological Association.

Zurbriggen, E. L., & Morgan, E. M. (2006). Who wants to marry a millionaire?: Reality dating television programs, attitudes toward sex, and sexual behaviors. *Sex Roles, 54,* 1–17.

Index

Page numbers followed by *f* indicate figures.

217